EMERGENCY CARE IN THE OPTOMETRIC SETTING

Notice

Medicine is an ever-changing science. As new research and clinical experience broaden our knowledge, changes in treatment and drug therapy are required. The authors and the publisher of this work have checked with sources believed to be reliable in their efforts to provide information that is complete and generally in accord with the standards accepted at the time of publication. However, in view of the possibility of human error or changes in medical sciences, neither the authors nor the publisher nor any other party who has been involved in the preparation or publication of this work warrants that the information contained herein is in every respect accurate or complete, and they disclaim all responsibility for any errors or omissions or for the results obtained from use of the information contained in this work. Readers are encouraged to confirm the information contained herein with other sources. For example and in particular, readers are advised to check the product information sheet included in the package of each drug they plan to administer to be certain that the information contained in this work is accurate and that changes have not been made in the recommended dose or in the contraindications for administration. This recommendation is of particular importance in connection with new or infrequently used drugs.

EMERGENCY CARE IN THE OPTOMETRIC SETTING

Michael H. Heiberger, OD, MA, FAAO
Associate Clinical Professor and
Instructor of Record for Emergency Care Courses
State College of Optometry
State University of New York
New York, New York

Richard J. Madonna, OD, MA, FAAO
Associate Professor and
Chief, Ocular Disease and Special Testing Service
State College of Optometry
State University of New York
New York, New York

Leon Nehmad, OD, FAAO
Assistant Clinical Professor
State College of Optometry
State University of New York
New York, New York

McGraw-Hill
Medical Publishing Division

New York   Chicago   San Francisco   Lisbon   London   Madrid   Mexico City   Milan
New Delhi   San Juan   Seoul   Singapore   Sydney   Toronto

Emergency Care in the Optometric Setting

1 2 3 4 5 6 7 8 9 0   DOC/DOC   0 9 8 7 6 5 4 3

ISBN 0-07-137553-8

This book was set in Minion by Westchester Book Composition.
The editors were Darlene Cooke and Lisa Silverman.
The production supervisor was Richard Ruzycka.
Project management was provided by Westchester Book Services.
The index was prepared by Schroeder Indexing Services.

This book is printed on acid-free paper.

Library of Congress Cataloging-in-Publication Data

Emergency care in the optometric setting / edited by Michael H. Heiberger,
    Richard J. Madonna, Leon Nehmad.—1st ed.
        p. ; cm.
    Includes bibliographical references and index.
    ISBN 0-07-137553-8
    1. Eye—Wounds and injuries.   2. Ophthalmologic emergencies.   3. Medical
emergencies.   4. Emergency medicine.   5. Optometry.   I. Heiberger,
Michael H.   II. Madonna, Richard J.   III. Nehmad, Leon.
    [DNLM: 1. Emergency Treatment—methods.   2. Eye Injuries—therapy.
3. Eye Diseases—therapy.   4. Optometry—methods. WW 525 E53 2004]
RE831.E533 2004
616.02'5'02461775—dc22

                                                                2003059256

CONTENTS

PREFACE

The optometrist of the twenty-first century is obliged to care for patients who suffer medical emergencies, be they general or ocular in nature. The vast majority of today's practicing optometrists have not been formally prepared in this area as part of their optometric education. Most have been educated in dealing with ocular emergencies as part of continuing education programs related to obtaining qualification for diagnostic and therapeutic pharmaceutical privileges. The very nature of the expanded scope and location of optometric practice increases the likelihood of the practitioner to be confronted with emergencies, either ocular or general. More optometrists are employed in hospital and other healthcare settings, where they care for more medically compromised patients. As well, more and more Medicare patients are being seen in optometric settings now that many optometric services are covered under that program.

During the early 1990s, the curriculum at SUNY College of Optometry was modified to include a 20-hour course in emergency care for students prior to their entering the clinical phase of the professional program at the beginning of their third year. Dr. Heiberger, the course coordinator, based the course on standardized American Red Cross courses in first aid and CPR and with the assistance of Drs. Madonna, Nehmad, and others, incorporated the practical aspects of caring for ocular emergencies that formerly existed in other parts of the curriculum. The course is more practical than theoretical in its approach. Materials prepared for this course form the basis for *Emergency Care in the Optometric Setting*, which is intended to serve as a manual/study guide for this and similar courses. The book is also intended as a ready reference for optometric practitioners in a variety of practice settings.

Part I deals with life-threatening medical emergencies that might confront the practicing optometrist. Preparedness for such emergencies is stressed in chapters on prevention, preparing the office environment and staff, and recognizing patients who have a high risk for experiencing these conditions. The basics of what to do for a patient suffering unconsciousness, breathing emergencies, chest pain, or sudden illness are presented. However, the book is not intended to be a substitute for formal training in first aid and CPR.

Part II provides specifics, in a very practical manner, on how optometrists should approach ocular urgencies and emergencies they may encounter according to how the patient presents. The intent is to provide a pragmatic and logical way of quickly assessing and managing ocular trauma, sudden diplopia, red eye, acute eye pain, flashes and floaters, and loss of vision. There is also a chapter on emergencies that may occur during postsurgical care. This section is designed to allow the practitioner to utilize it as a quick reference to key steps in the management of ocular emergencies as the patient is cared for. The material presented here is not intended as a replacement for more complete texts on the diagnosis, treatment, and management of these conditions.

The authors wish to thank their colleagues and students at the SUNY College of Optometry, from whom they learn every day.

Michael H. Heiberger
Richard J. Madonna
Leon Nehmad

Part I

LIFE-THREATENING EMERGENCIES

Chapter 1

Introduction

Life-threatening emergencies have been rare occurrences in the optometric setting. Both the increased scope of practice and the increase in the number of optometric patients who are elderly and/or medically compromised make it likely that the incidence of life-threatening episodes before, during, and after the optometric examination or procedure will increase. It is the purpose of this section to provide the optometrist with the knowledge and skills both to prevent such emergencies and to deal effectively with those life-threatening situations that cannot be avoided.

The U.S. Department of Health and Human Services lists heart disease as the nation's number one cause of death. In 1998, over 600,000 deaths were attributable to heart disease in the U.S. population for those over 65 years of age. The incidence of heart attacks is roughly twice the death rate. Thus well over 1 million U.S. citizens over the age of 65 will experience a life-threatening heart attack each year. This is but one of many potentially life-threatening emergencies that occur with increased frequency in this age group. Add to that the incidence of potentially life-threatening episodes in the younger age groups and one can see that there is a likelihood that the optometrist will encounter one or more life-threatening emergencies in the course of practice.

The fastest-growing segment of the population is the group over 80 years of age. This population has, as one would expect, a much larger percentage of medically compromised individuals. Often these individuals receive their eye care in institutional settings such as hospitals, nursing homes, and extended-care facilities. More and more optometrists are being employed in such facilities and, as health care professionals, are expected to be trained in the lifesaving skills necessary to provide immediate care in life-threatening situations. Certification in cardiopulmonary resuscitation (CPR) is usually a requirement for staff privileges in these facilities.

While the increase in the scope of optometric practice, such as the use of diagnostic and therapeutic pharmaceutical agents, has not increased the incidence of life-threatening emergencies in the optometric setting, it has had the effect of increasing the number of older patients seen by optometrists. This is as a result of Medicare coverage for conditions that, in the past, were outside the optometrist's scope of practice. The same holds true for patients covered under managed care contracts that offer medical eye care.

Even though the rationale for being prepared to deal with life-threatening emergencies lies within the optometrist's professional responsibility, it is probably more likely that the average optometrist will encounter life-threatening situations outside of his or her professional setting. Therefore, the knowledge and skills that the individual may gain in this area are more likely to be applied with family members, friends, relatives, or even strangers as opposed to patients. There is a far different consideration with regard to responsibility outside the office setting than there is in dealing with life-threatening emergencies that occur with patients.

There are many types of life-threatening emergencies as well as myriad causes for them. It is not the optometrist's responsibility to distinguish among these causes or to make any sort of medical differential diagnosis. Rather, it is his or her responsibility to keep the patient/victim alive until a person with a higher level of skill takes over. In legal parlance, the practitioner has a "duty to act" if a person under his or her care is the victim of a life-threatening emergency. In this regard, the optometrist, even though he or she has a duty to act in the optometric setting, is the equivalent of a first aid giver or "first responder" or "citizen responder," albeit with some formal certification in First Aid and CPR—unless, of course, the optometrist is also an emergency medical technician (EMT), a paramedic, or has some other higher level of training.

The broad categories of emergencies that will be dealt with in succeeding chapters include unconsciousness, breathing/respiratory emergencies, heart attacks, shock, and various other conditions of sudden illness such as diabetic emergencies, seizures, and strokes. Regardless of the type of emergency, it is the rescuer's primary responsibility to keep the victim alive and to assure that oxygenated blood is being circulated to the brain and other vital organs and that severe bleeding is controlled. There are various other conditions that may not be immediately life-threatening, but could become so, that the optometrist must be aware of. These include abnormal breathing, changes in skin color or moisture, and changes in awareness (Table 1–1).

It is not the purpose of this section to provide all of the knowledge and skills training that the optometrist must have in order to deal with life-threatening emergencies. It is, rather, to establish an awareness of what is involved in being prepared to deal with such emergencies and strongly to encourage optometrists to seek training and certification in life-saving skills for themselves and for others with whom they work. Many of the skills can only be learned by practicing them in the presence of a certified instructor. Once such

Table 1–1   Some Signs of Patients with
Possible Life-Threatening Conditions

Abnormal breathing
  Fast
  Slow
  Labored
  Shallow
Abnormal skin color
  Pale
  Bluish
  Red (flushed)
Abnormal skin moisture
  Sweating
Abnormal gait
  Staggering
  Unsteady
Abnormal expression
  Facial paralysis
  Facial tic
  Tremors
Chest pain

training and certification is secured, this book can then serve as a ready reference in the basics of providing emergency care.

The material in the chapters, in this section, dealing with each type of emergency is presented in an "as the patient presents" format in order to make it easier to locate the steps to take for each type of emergency described. Background information is included, as well, which provides the practitioner with a basic understanding of the physiology and causative factors for each type of emergency and suggestions about where to seek out additional information.

Chapter 2

Prevention

Preventing a medical emergency is always preferable to having to deal with one. Just as the practitioner should be concerned about public liability, such as avoiding dangerous conditions in the office, there should also be a concern about preventing, where at all possible, life-threatening medical emergencies from occurring in the professional setting. There is no question of potential public liability for such conditions as dangerous flooring or an icy sidewalk. Likewise, there is also an increased likelihood of a successful professional liability claim if a medical emergency could have been foreseen by the practitioner.

The practitioner has an opportunity, both in observing the patient and in the case history, to identify factors that may predispose a patient to having a medical emergency. In most such cases, the practitioner is alerted to the possibility and simply needs to pay increased attention to possible symptoms of such an emergency occurring during the optometric examination. For such patients, one might want to be cognizant of breathing rates, skin color, awareness, or other factors while performing optometric procedures. In other cases, the practitioner may wish to postpone the optometric examination until such time as the patient consults with a physician or until the examination can be conducted in an environment more suitable for dealing with possible medical emergencies.

OBSERVATION OF THE PATIENT

From the time the patient enters the office, the support staff, as well as the physician, should be aware of signs and symptoms that might indicate a medically compromised patient. The patient's previous record should alert the staff with regard to those conditions elicited during previous office visits. The office should consider some sort of medical alert coding on the face of the record such as a red tab or a red stamp with an indication of the nature of the patient's compromised medical condition.

Various signs that indicate that a patient might be prone to a life-threat-

Table 2–1 Factors in the Medical Case History That May Predispose Patients to a Possible Medical Emergency

Prior heart attack or other cardiac history
Drugs (legal and illegal)
Angina
Congestive heart failure (CHF)
Respiratory disease
  Asthma
  Bronchitis
  Chronic obstructive pulmonary disease (COPD)
  Other lung disease
Severe allergy
Seizures, fainting, or other episodes of unconsciousness
Prior stroke
Hypertension
Diabetes
Medications being taken for any of the above conditions

ening emergency are summarized (Table 2–1). Further discussion of the specific implications of these signs are discussed in succeeding chapters. Depending upon the nature of the sign exhibited, the patient's prior medical history, and/or discussion with the patient, a relative, or the patient's primary care physician, the optometrist may decide to proceed with the examination or to postpone it for a future date.

It is not logical that the optometrist make a differential diagnosis of the general medical problem. Even an emergency room physician, with sophisticated facilities and instrumentation, might take a long time to arrive at a cause for abnormal signs and symptoms. It is the responsibility of the optometrist to be sure that the patient is under the care of an appropriate physician as well as to deal with any medical emergency that might arise during the course of the patient's visit.

The signs listed in Table 1–1 must be considered as possible harbingers of life-threatening emergencies to the extent that they deviate from the normal *for that particular patient*. One should bear in mind that "normal" varies from individual to individual as well as for specific individuals with age.

Abnormal Breathing

Abnormality in the patient's breathing could be a sign of either a respiratory or circulatory disorder that could become life-threatening. The normal breathing rate is from 12 to 20 breaths per minute. Any significant variation from this rate is a signal that the patient may be medically compromised. Particularly fast and shallow breathing is indicative of a condition termed *hyperventilation*, which can be dealt with quite effectively in the office situation. The specific method is described in Chapter 6. Labored breathing, wherein the patient seems to be having difficulty with inspiration and expiration of breaths, is also indicative of a medically compromised patient.

Abnormal Skin Color

A patient whose skin appears pale, bluish, or red may be showing signs of a potentially life-threatening systemic condition. Pallor, or pale skin, or bluish skin is often indicative of a lack of oxygen being circulated to the cells of the body and this, in turn, suggests a serious respiratory or circulatory problem. Extreme redness of the skin can be from a number of causes, including hypertension and hyperthermia, which may be potentially life-threatening.

Abnormal Skin Moisture

Some perspiration in a patient, who may be apprehensive about the eye examination, can be expected. However, if the patient is sweating profusely in a normal or cool room, this may be an indication of a systemic condition that could become life-threatening. This is particularly true when sweating profusely is exhibited in combination with other signs or symptoms such as difficulty breathing or chest pain.

Abnormal Gait

If possible, it is often useful to observe the patient as he or she moves from the waiting room to the examining room. An unsteady or otherwise unusual gait could be indicative of an injured foot or ankle or it may be a sign of a medical problem of more general concern.

Abnormal Expression

A partial facial paralysis, even one that is barely noticeable, could be indicative of, for example, a mini-stroke that has gone undetected. Similarly, facial tics or tremors of the face or hands could indicate serious neurological problems. A patient who has had a previous stroke is much more prone to a subsequent stroke that may well be more extensive. While these patients may not suffer a medical emergency in the optometric office, it is best to refer them to an appropriate physician for a more complete diagnosis.

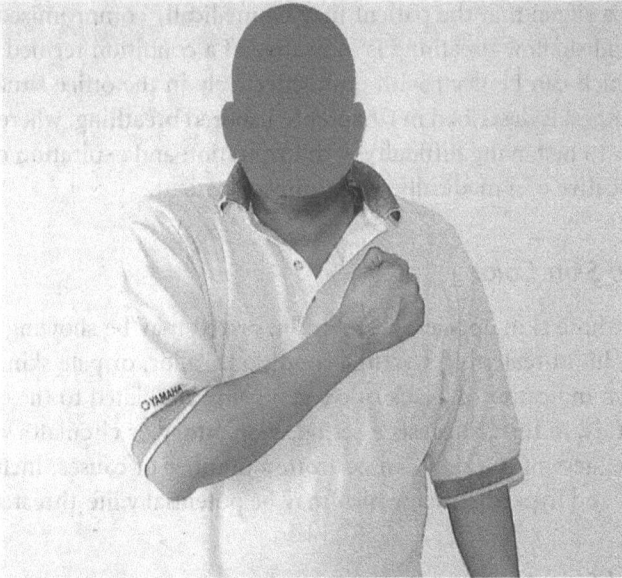

Figure 2–1. Levine's sign.

Chest Pain

Not all pain is potentially life-threatening. Angina, a generic term for chest pain, is a common symptom that does not necessarily mean that the patient is experiencing a heart attack. However, chest pain lasting for more than a few minutes should be considered as serious. The subject of dealing with patients who are experiencing chest pain is dealt with in detail in later chapters. In observing the patient, the optometrist should be aware of telltale signs of severe chest pain. These include grimacing and clutching at the chest. The latter, known as "Levine's sign," is almost always associated with a heart attack (Figure 2–1). Chest pain may not be reported as pain but rather as severe pressure, fullness, or squeezing in the center of the chest. If the patient reports that the feeling extends to the shoulders, neck, or arms and that he or she feels lightheaded, nauseous, or has difficulty breathing, assume that he or she is having a heart attack.

CASE HISTORY

The case history that the optometrist compiled at the beginning of any patient encounter typically includes a medical case history. The primary purpose of the medical case history is to determine what systemic conditions and related medications that the patient reports may have a bearing on the patient's visual status and ocular health. In addition, the optometrist is alerted to symptoms of medical problems that may require referral to a physician. It is also an opportunity for the optometrist to become aware of conditions that might produce life threatening emergencies (Table 2–1).

Eliciting information from the patient, prior to beginning any examination procedures, is valuable in learning about any past life-threatening emergencies that the patient may have experienced. It also provides an opportunity to find out about any medications that the patient is taking and the systemic conditions for which the patient may be under treatment, thereby alerting the optometrist to the increased possibility of a life-threatening emergency.

The legal principle of "foreseeability" is discussed in Chapter 10. Briefly stated, liability is increased if a life-threatening situation could have been foreseen and possibly prevented. This seems to be a paradox in that the diligent optometrist who takes a very complete medical history may end up in a more precarious legal position if a medical emergency actually occurs. However, this is not a good reason not to take a thorough case history, including a review of the patient's overall health and medications. If the optometrist, in his or her professional judgment, feels that the risk of a medical emergency occurring is great, postponement of the examination is then an option to consider. As no health practitioner can be sure when or whether a life-threatening emergency might occur, it is always best to be fully prepared and trained to deal with such emergencies.

There are several conditions that the optometrist should be familiar with that produce the vast majority of medical emergencies. A history of any of these conditions should alert the optometrist to be aware of signs and symptoms of a medical emergency that might develop during the examination. More detailed information about dealing with emergencies that arise from these conditions is dealt with in subsequent chapters.

Prior Heart Attack or Cardiac History

All known heart diseases can lead to cardiac arrest and sudden cardiac death. In fact, scarring from a prior heart attack is found in two-thirds of heart attack victims. Signs and symptoms of a heart attack should never be ignored in patients with a history of heart disease. Appropriate action should be taken immediately.

Drugs (Legal and Illegal)

Under certain conditions, various heart medications and other drugs—as well as illegal drug abuse—can lead to abnormal heart rhythms that cause sudden death. The optometrist needs to be particularly alert to signs and symptoms that signal a heart attack in patients using these substances.

Angina

A patient with a history of angina, or mild to moderate chest pain, may experience this symptom during the optometric examination. Such a patient will usually have medication (nitroglycerin tablets) with them that should alleviate the pain within minutes. If it does not, the practitioner should treat the patient as if he or she were having a heart attack.

Congestive Heart Failure

Congestive heart failure (or CHF or heart failure) is a condition in which the heart cannot pump enough blood to meet the needs of the body's other organs. This can result from a variety of causes including high blood pressure, coronary artery disease, or other heart disease. Patients with heart failure cannot exert themselves because they have shortness of breath and become easily tired. The optometrist should be aware that patients with CHF may exhibit breathing difficulty during the optometric examination. In rare cases, fluid can accumulate quickly in the lungs. This condition, known as acute pulmonary edema, is very serious and can be fatal.

Respiratory Disease

More than 17 million Americans suffer from asthma, including almost 5 million under the age of 18. Chronic obstructive pulmonary disease (COPD, chronic bronchitis, and emphysema) afflicts another 17 million Americans. These and other forms of lung disease, including lung cancer, can cause a respiratory emergency in the office.

Severe Allergy

A wide variety of things can cause an anaphylactic reaction, or a severe allergic reaction, including food, with peanuts and shellfish being the most common, although any food can be responsible. Drugs such as penicillin and vaccines are common causes, as are insect stings from wasps, bees, or hornets. Any substance has the potential for causing a life-threatening allergy.

Seizures, Fainting, or Other Episodes of Unconsciousness

Regardless of cause, unconsciousness is always potentially life-threatening. Patients with a history of unconsciousness, with or without known cause, are more likely to experience such episodes than those who do not have such a history.

Prior Stroke

As with patients who have had prior instances of unconsciousness, patients with a prior history of stroke are more prone to subsequent strokes. The optometrist needs to be aware of the signs and symptoms of stroke as they may occur without the patient losing consciousness.

Hypertension

Medical emergencies due to hypertension are rare. However, patients with a history of hypertension often have associated medical conditions that may increase the chances that a medical emergency could occur. In cases of severe, or malignant, hypertension (diastolic pressure above 115 *or* systolic above 200 when the diastolic is above 90), there is a significantly increased risk of a medical emergency and these patients should be immediately referred to an emergency room facility.

Diabetes

Diabetics are susceptible to two types of medical emergencies, diabetic coma and insulin shock. The former is a condition induced by insufficient insulin and the latter usually occurs when the patient has self-administered insulin, or another diabetic medication, and forgotten to eat. This latter condition is remedied by oral administration of sugar. Diabetics usually carry candy, or some form of easily administered sugar, for this purpose. Paradoxically, treatment of diabetic coma is exactly the same. The reason for this is that one cannot easily distinguish between diabetic coma and insulin shock.

Medications Being Taken for Any of the Above Conditions

In eliciting information concerning medications, it is important for the optometrist to determine the condition for which the patient is taking each particular medication. Medications that are commonly used to treat certain specific conditions may also be used less frequently to treat different conditions for which the medication is also approved or not approved ("off-label use"). Knowing the specific medical condition(s) for which the patient is being treated helps to alert the optometrist to the potential of a medical emergency.

SAFETY ISSUES IN THE OPTOMETRIC SETTING

No discussion of prevention would be complete without considering factors that could lead to accidental life-threatening emergencies in the optometrist's office. Accidents are a leading cause of injury, subsequent illness, and death, particularly in the elderly. Safety in the optometric setting should be a concern, not only for patients, but also for those who accompany the patient, as well as for the staff. While it is not the purpose of this text to offer advice on office design or other environmental concerns, it is important for the optometrist to be aware of environmental factors that relate to safety and to the general health of those who work in or come to that setting for care (Table 2–2).

Floor Coverings

Care should be taken to avoid slippery floors, loose carpeting, thresholds, or other floor-level obstacles that could cause someone to fall or lose his or her balance. A change in floor surface, as, for example, from carpeting in a hallway to a tiled floor in the examination room, may cause a patient with already impaired balance to stagger or fall.

Lighting

Optometrists, in particular, should have an awareness of the importance of adequate lighting to a patient's overall vision. Not only should all reception and work areas have adequate lighting, but care should be taken to have the examination room fully lit when the patient makes the transition from the re-

Table 2–2 Environmental Safety Factors in the Optometric Setting

Floor coverings
Lighting
Color
Placement of furniture
Examination equipment
Ventilation

ception area. If the optometrist, or other staff, must leave the patient alone in the examination room, the room lighting should be turned on until the staff person returns to continue the examination procedure.

Color

The color of the walls, floor, ceiling, and furnishings can be a safety factor. For example, there should be color contrast that permits visually impaired patients to discern transitions from space to space within the office and to distinguish furnishings from background. A good professional interior designer can be of help in this regard.

Placement of Furniture

Careful attention to the placement of office furnishings and to traffic patterns within the office is important in addressing safety concerns. A diabetic patient who is there for a dilated fundus examination may get into serious medical difficulty if he or she bangs a leg on a chair and creates a wound that could be slow to heal and susceptible to severe infection due to the diabetes.

Examination Equipment

Safety within the examination room is extremely important, particularly because of the low level of room lighting often required when performing optometric procedures. Care should be taken when assisting the patient into and out of the examination chair. When pieces of equipment are not in use, they should be moved to a position where the patient cannot be injured when getting out of the chair. When examining a patient using auxiliary equipment that requires that the patient be seated on a stool or movable chair, care should be taken to make sure wheels are locked and that the patient is supported by another individual while the optometrist or technician is performing the procedure.

Ventilation

For patients who have respiratory problems, it is particularly important that there be good air circulation and properly maintained temperature and humidity. Air filtration is important in preventing problems for patients with allergies to dust or pollen or who have a history of asthma.

Chapter **3**

The In-Office Emergency

In this and in subsequent chapters, potentially life-threatening emergencies will be discussed as they may present to the optometrist. Step-by-step care of each emergency will also be presented. However, it is not intended that these regimens replace the skills and procedures taught in emergency care courses given by such agencies as the American Red Cross and the American Heart Association. Formal training of optometrists and their office staff members is discussed in Chapter 9.

It is important to remember that the optometrist, when confronted with a patient experiencing a life-threatening emergency, is going to treat the symptoms and not the disease. The specific disease entity causing the life-threatening signs or symptoms may not be known. Nor is it important to know the diagnosis in order to provide immediate effective care. It will be left to the physician, usually in the emergency room, to follow up in determining the cause.

EMERGENCIES OUTSIDE OF THE EXAMINATION ROOM

Before considering emergencies that might occur during the optometric examination, let us first discuss patients, or even accompanying relatives or friends, who might experience a medical emergency in some part of the office other than the examination room. This would most likely be the waiting or reception room. Even though emergencies could occur elsewhere such as in restrooms, dispensary, or hallways, the waiting or reception room is the place where patients spend most of their time when not in the examination room proper.

Most office designs allow for the reception area to be visible by office staff. It is common in many offices, however, for there to be a glass window partitioning the business office from the reception area. Not only is it good practice management for office staff to be visible and audible to patients and vice

17

Table 3–1   Recognizing an Emergency in the Office

Look for unusual sights or behaviors
Listen for peculiar sounds
Be aware of uncommon odors

---

versa, it is also an important safety factor. This will be discussed in more detail later in Chapter 9.

Before anyone can react to an emergency, he or she must recognize that an emergency exists. This includes recognition that an individual is experiencing a medical emergency as well as environmental factors that could lead to a medical emergency such as leaking gas, fire, or extremes of temperature (Table 3–1).

The following steps apply in all circumstances, outside the examination room, in the examination room, or even out of the office. Remember, however, that if it is a patient experiencing a medical emergency while being examined or treated, the optometrist must render appropriate care. There is no choice. It is prudent, however, for the optometrist, and other office staff, to be prepared to render care for anyone, anywhere on the premises, who suffers a life-threatening medical emergency.

RECOGNIZING AN EMERGENCY IN THE OFFICE

Look for Unusual Signs or Behaviors

Patient unusually quiet—*Is he asleep or has he lost consciousness?*

Patient appears confused or drowsy or slurs speech—*Is this normal for this patient?*

Patient clutches chest or throat—*Could this be a sign of difficulty breathing or severe pain?*

Patient unusually restless—*Has the patient just been waiting too long or is something wrong?*

Patient's skin pale or flushed or sweaty—*Is this more than pre-exam jitters?*

Listen for Peculiar Sounds

Thud or other loud noise—*Did the patient fall or collapse?*

Wheezing, noisy or labored breathing—*Does the patient seem distressed?*

Be Aware of Uncommon Odors

Strange odor on patient's breath—*Is this poor oral hygiene or could it be the sign of a diabetic emergency?*

Smell of natural gas—*In a closed environment, a gas leak could lead to unconsciousness or, worse yet, an explosion.*

Smoke—*Can often be smelled before it can be seen. Where there's smoke . . .*

EMERGENCIES IN THE EXAMINATION ROOM

There are certain environmental factors in the examination room that, if attended to, can help to prevent emergencies from occurring, make them less severe if they do occur, and make them easier to deal with. Some of these factors that relate to office design are discussed in Chapter 2. The following are some general considerations with prevention in mind:

In and Out of the Chair

It is often difficult and sometimes awkward, particularly for elderly patients, to maneuver themselves into or out of the examination chair. The optometrist should assist the patient both at the beginning and at the end of the examination by gently guiding the patient into and out of the chair and positioning him- or herself so as to catch the patient if he or she should stumble. When not using equipment that is attached to the examining stand, be sure it is placed in a position where it is not possible for the patient to come into contact with it when sitting down in the examining chair or getting up from it.

Don't Leave the Patient in the Dark

If it is necessary to leave the examination room, turn on lights so as not to leave the patient in a darkened room. A patient attempting to get out of the chair when the lights are out is a candidate for a potential injury due to a fall. It is also a good idea to have full lighting on in the examination room when the patient is entering or leaving.

Don't Lock Yourself Out

If the examination room door has a lock on it, make sure it is not engaged when you leave the room. Not only is it embarrassing for the patient to have to let you back in, it could be dangerous for some patients with impaired mobility.

FIRST CONSIDERATIONS FOR A MEDICAL EMERGENCY IN THE EXAMINATION ROOM

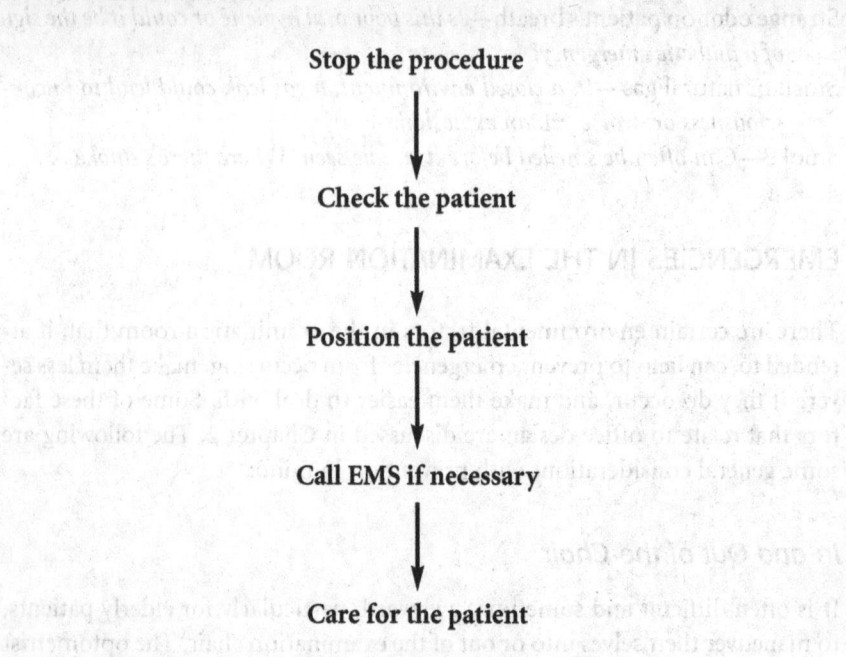

Stop the procedure

↓

Check the patient

↓

Position the patient

↓

Call EMS if necessary

↓

Care for the patient

Stop the Procedure

This may seem obvious. However, the optometrist is often so intent on resolving the patient's visual problem that the signs of a potentially life-threatening medical emergency may go unrecognized or, if recognized, may not get the immediate attention that is required.

Check the Patient

Checking the patient is necessary in order to determine whether or not the patient is conscious, whether there is breathing, and whether there is a pulse. Treatment of the patient depends on what is found. Specific treatment for each condition will be discussed in succeeding chapters.

Position the Patient

If the patient is conscious, he or she should be placed in the most comfortable position for the patient. This is usually the position where the patient can breathe most easily. It is usually best to leave the patient in the chair. If the patient is unconscious, it may be necessary to reposition the patient in order to fully assess his or her condition. This may often be done by tilting the examination chair all the way back thus alleviating the need to move the patient out of the chair. As we will see later, there are situations where it may be necessary to move the patient onto the floor in order to provide a firm surface for procedures such as chest compressions (part of CPR).

Call the Emergency Medical System (EMS) if Necessary

How to call EMS is discussed in Chapter 5. Whether to call EMS is sometimes a judgment call. The optometrist would rather avoid a team of paramedics or emergency medical technicians rushing into the office. However, the optometrist's first consideration is the patient with the life-threatening emergency and the most important thing that can be done for that patient is to call EMS.

Care for the Patient

The succeeding chapters discuss the appropriate care for each type of emergency. The type of emergency, and how it is treated, is determined by what is found when checking the patient. In many of the emergencies described, care for the patient includes the provision of basic life support. This consists of monitoring airway, breathing, and circulation (the ABCs) and providing the care indicated by the assessment of these functions. Such care might include clearing the airway, rescue breathing, cardiopulmonary resuscitation, or automated defibrillation. These procedures are described in succeeding chapters.

Chapter 4

Checking the Patient

The first consideration in responding to an emergency is to determine if it is safe for the rescuer to approach the victim. In cases of fire, smoke, downed electrical wires, or noxious fumes, it may not be safe to render care until the dangerous condition is addressed. It is usually not wise to risk the rescuer becoming another victim. Within the optometric setting and, particularly during the examination, safety of the rescuer is usually not an issue. The steps to follow will vary depending on whether or not the patient is conscious.

CHECKING A CONSCIOUS PATIENT

1. Be aware of signs or symptoms of an emergency such as abnormal breathing, lightheadedness, confusion, or pain.
2. Help the patient into a comfortable position. Depending on the nature of the symptoms, this may be from fully upright to fully supine in the examination chair.
3. While calming the patient, inquire as to the nature of the symptoms and whether or not they have ever occurred before.
4. Treat according to what is found.*
5. Call EMS if necessary.

CHECKING AN UNCONSCIOUS PATIENT

1. Be sure that the patient is really unconscious. It has not been unknown for patients to fall asleep during an examination. The best way to establish unconsciousness is to:

---

*Descriptions of, and the treatment for, specific medical emergencies are described in the following chapters according to what is found when checking the patient.

    ○ tap the patient's shoulders vigorously enough to be felt but not hard enough to exacerbate or cause a neck injury

    ○ shout into the patient's ear, being loud enough to awaken even a deep sleeper

If the patient responds, proceed as with a conscious patient. If there is no response, assume that the patient is unconscious and proceed to step #2.

2. Once it is determined that an adult patient is unconscious and that the episode is not a simple fainting spell, EMS should be called immediately. An office staff person, an individual accompanying the patient, or anyone else for that matter should be directed to call. If no one else is available, the optometrist must place the call. For a child or infant, it is recommended that a minute or so of care be given first prior to leaving the patient to go and call.

3. Position the patient so that the patient's condition can be properly assessed. In all likelihood, this would involve easing the patient to the floor on his or her back. If the examination space allows, it may be possible to tend to the patient while he or she is fully reclined in the examination chair. However, if chest compressions should become necessary, the patient would most likely have to be moved to the floor.

4. The patient should be assessed with regard to the ABCs (Airway, Breathing, and Circulation).

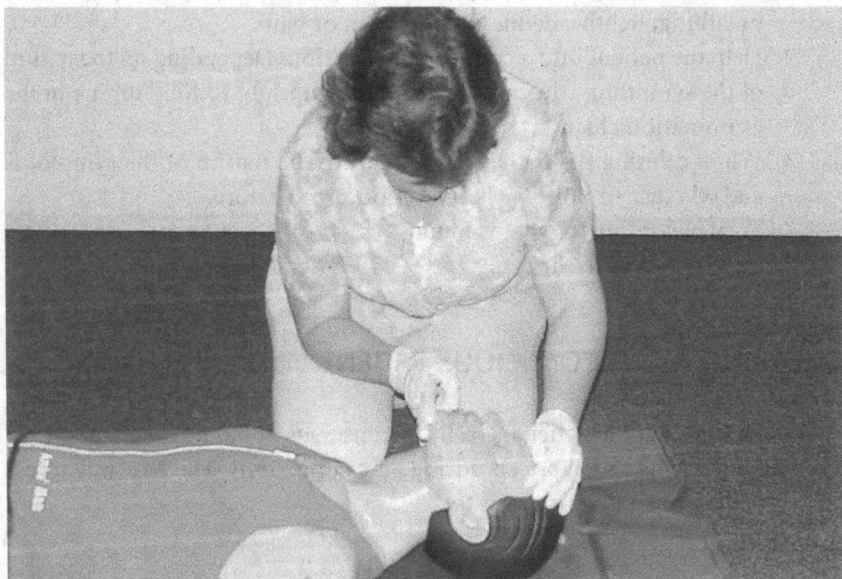

Figure 4–1. Opening the airway.

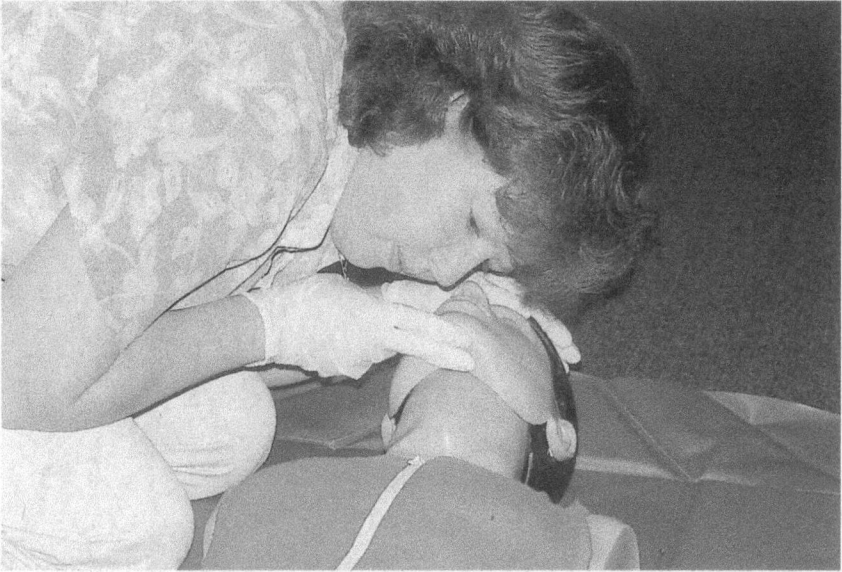

Figure 4–2. Looking, listening, and feeling for breathing.

○ Open the airway by lifting the chin and tilting the victim's forehead (Figure 4–1).
○ Look, listen, and feel for breathing for five seconds. It is necessary to have your ear very close to the patient's nose and mouth and to keep your eyes on the patient's chest (Figure 4–2). You can then, "look, listen, and feel for breathing."
○ If there is breathing, simply monitor the patient and wait for EMS. If there is no breathing, give two slow breaths. Breathing into a patient and the use of various breathing devices are discussed later.
○ Check the carotid pulse for 5 to 10 seconds.
○ Treat according to what is found.

It is very important that the optometrist maintain current certification in rendering emergency care at the first aid level through taking formal courses. This is discussed in Chapter 9.

Chapter 5

Unconsciousness

Unconsciousness, regardless of the cause, can be potentially life-threatening. Likewise, the steps to follow in dealing with an unconscious individual are the same regardless of what caused the person to become unconscious. Over 30 causes of unconsciousness have been identified in the medical literature. Therefore, a differential diagnosis of this condition in the optometrist's office is both impossible and not necessary in order to provide emergency first aid to a victim who is unconscious.

The most common cause of unconsciousness, and the one that the optometrist will most likely encounter, is vasopressor syncope, also known as the "common faint." Fortunately, it is also one of the least serious forms of unconsciousness. The longer the patient remains unconscious, however, the more serious the incident is. If a patient has a history of fainting, the optometrist should be alert to a recurrence during the examination. Often the stress, the shining of lights in the patient's eyes, or other factors inherent in an optometric examination will cause a patient who is prone to fainting to do just that. This type of fainting is usually not serious and the patient regains consciousness within five minutes of being placed in a supine position. If he or she does not, the situation can be considered a medical emergency and the Emergency Medical Services (EMS) system should be activated.

Unconsciousness is much more serious when the patient has labored breathing or is not breathing at all or has no pulse. Dealing with these situations, on a step-by-step basis, will be discussed in later chapters. There are, however, some general considerations about dealing with an unconscious patient. *The most important thing you can do for an unconscious patient is to call the EMS system.*

CALLING EMS

It sounds simple! Call 911! Unless the call is made appropriately, however, valuable time may be lost and this lost time may well make the difference between

Table 5–1   Factors to Consider in Calling EMS

Who should call?
Using the most appropriate emergency phone number
Using a mobile phone
Information needed
Following the "script"
Directing the ambulance

life and death. The factors discussed here apply to calling EMS whether or not the patient is conscious. However, as part of the information given to the EMS operator, it is vital to report that the patient is unconscious if this is in fact the case. It may well hasten the response time.

There are a number of factors to consider when calling EMS (Table 5–1).

Who Should Call?

If there is more than one person on the scene, the individual with the highest level of training should take charge. The optometrist taking care of the patient, in his or her office setting, is the most likely person to take charge and should direct a specific individual to call 911 or the appropriate emergency number. It is important not just to say, "Somebody call an ambulance!" Rather, he or she should say, "You, call an ambulance," while pointing to a specific individual or, better yet, something like, "You, Susie, call an ambulance!"

Using the Most Appropriate Emergency Phone Number

The use of 911 is not yet universal. Many smaller communities, and even some cities, use a phone number other than 911 to activate the EMS system in their locality. It is important to know that number *both* for the community in which you work and for the community in which you live. These numbers, along with other emergency numbers, are listed in the front pages of your local phone directory. Local EMS or volunteer ambulance services often provide stickers or magnets with their emergency phone number.

Time is of the essence when calling to activate an EMS response. Even a minute or two could make the difference between life and death or irreversible loss of function. Many areas that have 911 emergency phone service either utilize that service for all emergencies (fire, police, and ambulance) or utilize 911 on a region-wide or county-wide basis with a central communications center. In either instance, the call must be transferred to the ambulance service for the particular locality where emergency assistance is required. This takes time. Knowing the direct number to the agency that operates the ambulances in the local community (EMS service, fire department, or volunteer ambulance) saves time.

Using a Mobile Phone

The use of mobile or cellular phones has made emergency calling much more readily accessible, particularly away from the home or office. There are two considerations that are necessary when using mobile phones to call for an ambulance.

Depending on your location and the type of service that the phone is utilizing, the caller, when dialing 911, may or may not reach the correct EMS or ambulance service for the locality where help is needed. If a standard phone is readily available, it may be a better choice since many emergency response agencies have equipment that can detect the caller's phone number and address electronically.

A second important consideration is to know your own mobile phone number. You should be able to give that number to the emergency operator so that you can be recontacted.

Information Needed

There is certain information that is vital for the caller to have when making an emergency call for an ambulance. The following information is vital in getting the fastest and most appropriate response.

1. Location of the incident. This should include the address as well as the floor and room number.
2. Nature of the emergency. This is important to the emergency operator in knowing what type of assistance to send as well as in the triage of emergency calls. An unconscious victim, for example, would most likely have priority over a conscious victim.
3. Number of victims. This is important in situations such as motor vehicle accidents where multiple ambulances may be needed.

Following the "Script"

Most emergency operators utilize a script or a set of prepared questions that are followed in sequence to determine how to prioritize their calls and to assess each individual situation so that the proper help is dispatched. This also helps the operator to provide instructions, over the phone, about what to do until help arrives. This is particularly valuable where the caller and/or the would-be rescuer is not trained in providing emergency care.

Often, to the caller, it seems as if the emergency operator is wasting time and asking a lot of needless questions. It is important to answer all the questions as they are asked. This scripting, or rote manner in which information is communicated, has usually been developed as the result of years of experience in handling emergency calls. It is the best way to obtain information under stressful circumstances and the caller should be patient and answer as quickly and accurately as possible.

In order to be sure that all of the emergency operator's questions have been answered, the caller should not hang up until the operator does.

Directing the Ambulance

The person making the call, or another specifically designated individual, should position him- or herself so as to be seen by the approaching ambulance. This makes it possible to direct ambulance personnel to the victim quickly and by the most direct route.

Chapter **6**

Breathing Emergencies

If a patient stops breathing, permanent brain damage begins to occur within four to six minutes and cardiac arrest occurs within 5 to 10 minutes. In most cases, an ambulance will not respond in time to prevent these consequences of oxygen deprivation. The patient's blood must be kept oxygenated and, if the heart stops beating, the oxygenated blood must be kept flowing to the brain and other vital organs by the use of chest compressions.

BREATHING EMERGENCIES—CONSCIOUS PATIENT

It is, of course, best to deal with a breathing emergency *before* the patient stops breathing. There are several conditions that are considered breathing emergencies in which the patient is conscious but is having difficulty breathing. These conditions include asthma, hyperventilation, congestive heart failure, and acute pulmonary edema.

Asthma

Asthma may be an allergic or nonallergic reaction that results in narrowing of the airways (trachea and bronchi). Its incidence is about 5% in adults and up to 10% in children. In addition to allergens, both physiological and psychological stress may bring on an acute attack. In the acute attack the patient has difficulty breathing, has a feeling of suffocation, and may have a tightness across the chest. A sign unique to asthma is "nasal flaring."

Most asthmatics carry with them a bronchodilator in the form of an aerosol inhaler containing a sympathomimetic or an anticholinergic agent. Assist the patient in locating the inhaler and, if necessary, in administering the bronchodilator agent. This will usually ameliorate the acute attack. If it does not, EMS personnel should be summoned.

31

In summary, if a patient exhibits signs of an acute asthmatic episode:

Place the patient in a comfortable position (fully or partially upright)

↓

Keep calm and calm the patient

↓

Locate the bronchodilator and, if necessary, assist the patient to administer it

↓

If several doses do not relieve symptoms, summon EMS personnel

↓

Provide basic life support

Hyperventilation

Hyperventilation is an increased rate and/or depth of respiration and its most common cause is anxiety. The normal rate of respiration for an adult is 12–20 breaths per minute. A rate of 25 or above may be considered as hyperventilation. The condition causes a decrease in carbon dioxide that results in chemical changes in the blood that may cause a feeling of lightheadedness. This is a condition that can best be prevented by calming an anxious patient before beginning the examination.

The most effective treatment for hyperventilation is to have the patient breathe into a paper (not plastic) bag. When a patient rebreathes his or her own exhaled air, the carbon dioxide concentration in the patient's blood is increased and normal breathing restored. The paper bag is held gently over the nose and mouth while the patient is encouraged to breathe slowly. If a paper bag is not available, having the patient breathe into his or her own cupped hands is an alternative. In the rare instances where rebreathing exhaled air is not effective, 10–15 mg of diazepam may be administered intravenously, intramuscularly, or orally depending on which route of administration is available to the optometrist.

Steps in caring for a patient who is hyperventilating:

Place the patient in a comfortable position

↓

Keep calm and calm the patient

↓

Have patient breathe into a paper bag or into cupped hands

↓

Administer diazepam (if needed)

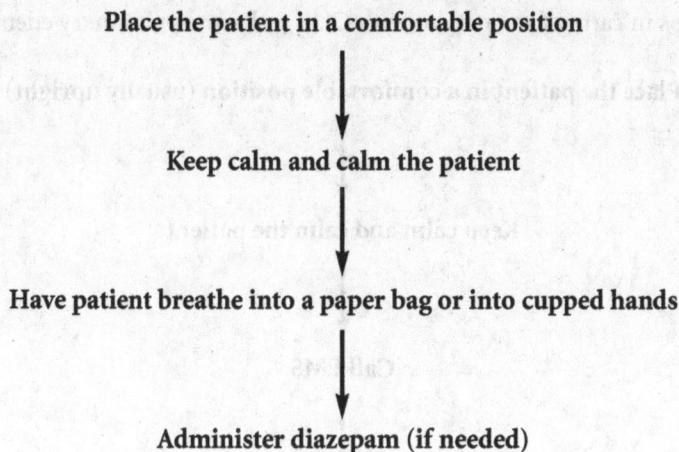

Congestive Heart Failure (CHF) and Acute Pulmonary Edema

Congestive heart failure (CHF) refers to fluid accumulating in the pulmonary circulation and lungs as well as systemically. Failure of the left side of the heart produces respiratory distress while failure of the right side of the heart causes systemic blood vessels and capillaries to retain fluid and results in peripheral edema. CHF rarely results in an office emergency. However, a sudden rapid filling of the lungs with fluid can cause a life-threatening condition known as acute pulmonary edema.

CHF is a common affliction in the United States. Nearly 2 million people exhibit the signs and symptoms of this condition, which is almost always associated with heart disease. Signs and symptoms include shortness of breath (particularly in the supine position and upon exertion), swelling of the ankles, skin pallor, sweating, general weakness, hyperventilation, and wheezing. A distinctive characteristic of CHF is the prominence of the jugular veins in the neck even in the upright position. These patients may be taking diuretics and/or vasodilators or inotropic agents such as digoxin. Patients with signs and symptoms of CHF will not usually require emergency care but should be monitored during the examination for worsening of these signs or symptoms.

The key issue for optometrists is to identify patients with CHF by observation, and in the case history, and to exercise care during the examination to relieve stress and to prevent the onset of acute pulmonary edema. Severe symptoms, indicative of acute pulmonary edema, such as subjective shortness of breath even at rest, wheezing, cyanosis (bluish skin), extreme anxiety, moist rales upon auscultation of the lungs, and frothy pink sputum should be treated as a medical emergency and EMS personnel should be summoned.

Steps in caring for a patient with CHF and acute pulmonary edema:

Place the patient in a comfortable position (usually upright)

↓

Keep calm and calm the patient

↓

Call EMS

↓

Provide basic life support

Conscious Choking

While not commonly encountered during the examination, a person with an obstructed airway requires immediate attention. This type of emergency, if encountered in the office, is more likely to occur in the reception room and is often the result, in adults, of food lodged in the trachea or, in children, of food or other objects that obstruct the intake of air. An individual unable to cough, speak, or breathe has an obstructed airway. A high-pitched wheezing sound can also be considered a sign of an obstructed airway. If the person can cough or talk, he or she does not have an obstructed airway and should be encouraged to keep coughing until the partial obstruction is cleared. *Do not slap the person on the back.*

In the case of an obstructed airway, EMS should be called as soon as possible.

The intervention required for a conscious choking individual is a technique commonly known as the Heimlich maneuver (Figure 6–1). This is an effective way of dislodging an object by giving abdominal thrusts. Note that the technique is different for an infant (below one year of age) and consists of abdominal thrusts and back blows while holding the infant upside down.

In the case where the rescuer cannot get his or her arms around an obese person or where the victim is pregnant and abdominal thrusts are too dangerous, chest thrusts should be substituted. In all cases, if the victim is not the patient, permission must be given in order to help. If permission is not given, wait a few minutes and the victim will fall to the floor unconscious and then permission is implied and help can be rendered.

The steps in caring for a conscious choking victim are summarized in Table 6–1.

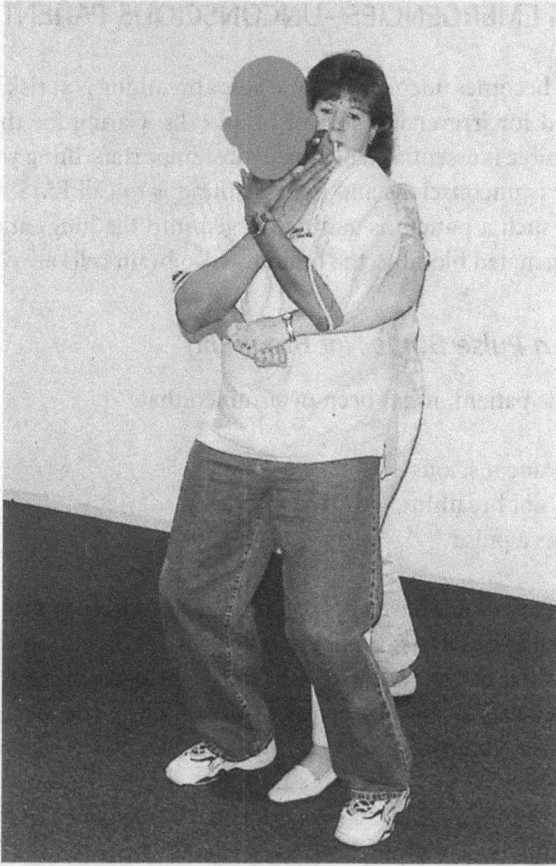

Figure 6–1. The Heimlich maneuver.

Table 6–1 Caring for a Conscious Choking
Adult or Child (over one year of age)

Get permission to help (if not your patient)
Have someone call EMS
With victim standing, move behind victim
Position fists for abdominal thrusts
Give sharp inward and upward thrusts until the object is dislodged,
   the victim becomes unconscious, or EMS personnel arrive

BREATHING EMERGENCIES—UNCONSCIOUS PATIENT

A patient who becomes unconscious and stops breathing is at risk both for cardiac arrest and for irreversible loss of brain cells. Caring for that person as quickly as possible is essential. The single most important thing you can do for a patient who is unconscious and not breathing is to call EMS. The primary concern with such a patient is getting oxygen into the lungs and circulating sufficient oxygenated blood to the brain to keep brain cells alive.

Patient Has a Pulse But Is Not Breathing

In checking the patient, it has been determined that:

The patient is unconscious
The patient is not breathing
The patient has a pulse

After the patient has been checked and EMS has been summoned, rescue breathing should be started as quickly as possible. A breathing device such as a face mask or bag-valve mask (see Chapter 9) helps to make rescue breathing more efficient but mouth-to-mouth breathing is effective. It is natural to be concerned about disease transmission and this is also discussed in Chapter 9.

Rescue breathing (Table 6–2) is performed by making a tight seal around the patient's mouth while pinching the patient's nostrils shut (Figure 6–2). With effective breaths, the patient's chest should rise and fall. For an adult patient, 12 breaths per minute (one every five seconds) should be administered; for a child or infant it is 20 breaths per minute (one every three seconds). The pulse should be rechecked after the first minute and every few minutes after that as the heart may stop due to lack of oxygen.

Table 6–2 Rescue Breathing

Check for unconsciousness
Call EMS
Position patient on a flat surface
Check ABCs (Airway, Breathing, Circulation)
If the patient is not breathing, but has a pulse:
    Give one breath every 5 seconds
    Recheck pulse after 1 minute and every few minutes thereafter

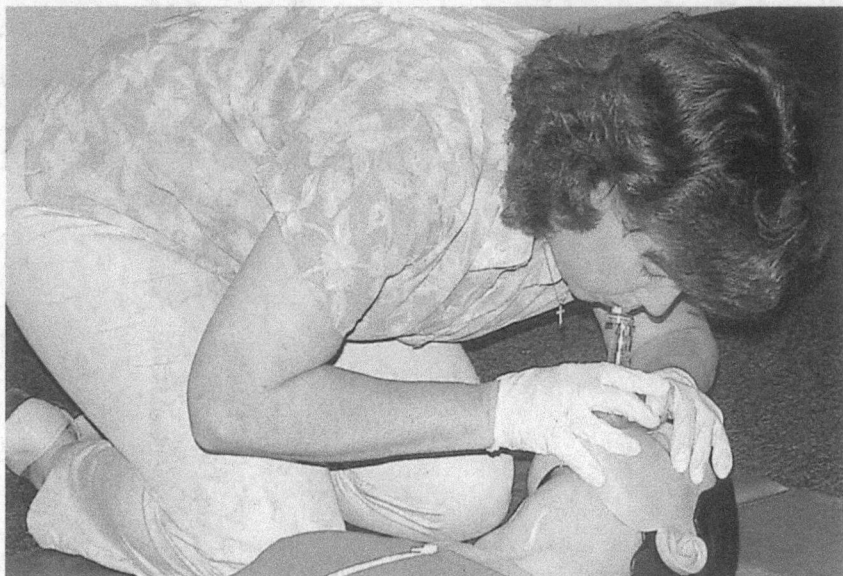

Figure 6-2. Rescue breathing using a pocket face mask.

Once begun, rescue breathing should continue until:

1. EMS personnel arrive and take over, or
2. another rescuer arrives and takes over, or
3. the victim begins to breathe on his or her own, or
4. the rescuer is too exhausted to continue, or
5. there is no pulse (go to CPR and/or defibrillation).

Unconscious Choking Patient

When checking an unconscious patient (see Chapter 4), the two slow breaths will not go in. In this situation, assume that the *airway is obstructed*. Often, tilting the head and lifting the jaw is enough to open the airway. Therefore, if breaths do not go in, the head should be carefully retilted and breaths tried again. If breaths still do not go in, give 15 chest compressions, do a finger sweep if an object is seen, and try again to get two breaths in. The proper position for chest compressions is illustrated in Figure 6-3. *It is strongly advised that chest compressions not be attempted unless one has taken a course in CPR.* Once the object is cleared and breaths go in, continue with checking the ABCs.

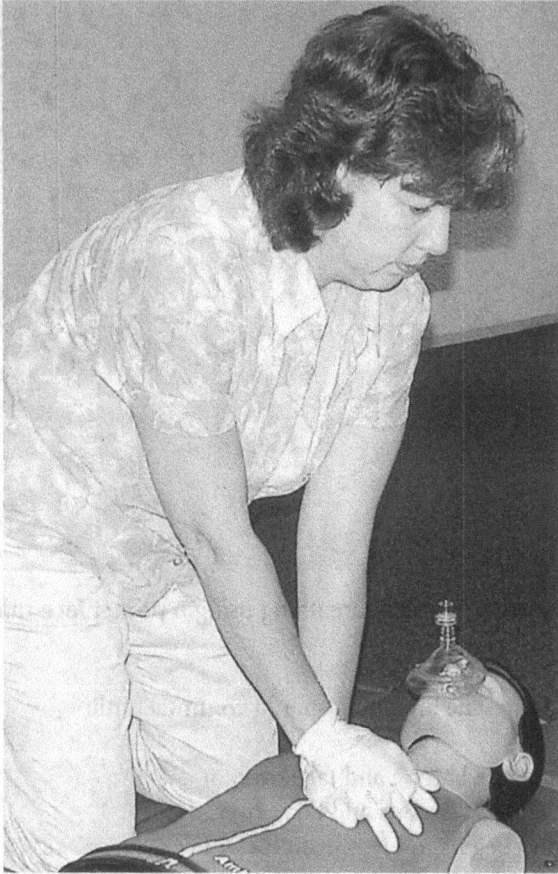

Figure 6–3. Proper position for chest compressions.

Special Situations

1. Stomas—A patient who has had surgery in the neck or throat area may be breathing through a tube in the neck known as a stoma. To give breaths to such a patient, one must breathe into the stoma rather than the mouth.
2. Dentures—If a patient is wearing dentures, they should be left in place. It is easier then to get a good seal around the patient's mouth.
3. Vomiting—If a patient vomits, his or her head should be turned to the side and any material in the mouth swept out before proceeding.

Chapter 7

Sudden Illness

A variety of systemic conditions with a variety of causes can account for a patient exhibiting signs of illness before, during, or after the optometric examination. In these instances, it is less important to render specific care than it is to promptly summon EMS personnel. It may not be possible for the optometrist to determine quickly what the specific illness is. Moreover, rapidly getting the patient into the care of more advanced medical personnel may be essential in saving the patient's life or, at the least, minimizing any permanent loss or disability as a result of the acute episode.

The case history is important in alerting the practitioner to the possibility of episodes of sudden illness. Patients with a history of sudden illness may also be wearing a medical alert tag.

Notwithstanding the above, several major conditions that may cause episodes of sudden illness are discussed here along with the recommended first aid treatment for these conditions to be applied while awaiting the arrival of EMS personnel. This is not a complete listing of such conditions but rather constitutes those conditions that the optometrist might be most likely to encounter.

SEIZURE

Patients who exhibit the signs of a seizure (generally seen as convulsions) are usually not in a life-threatening situation even though they may look like they are. Though such patients do become unconscious, it is usually for a short period of time. Recurrent seizure activity, or epilepsy, has an incidence of one in 200 individuals. The case history should elicit which patients have had a history of seizures. Such patients are often being maintained medically on one or more antiepileptic drugs, the most common being Dilantin.

In most cases, the tonic-clonic convulsions will cease within a few minutes and the patient will regain consciousness. The seizure may even be followed by a period of sleep. As a rule of thumb, EMS should be called for seizures lasting more than five minutes or for repeated seizures.

The most important thing that the optometrist can do for a patient experiencing a seizure is to make sure that the patient does not injure him- or herself. *Do not* place anything in the patient's mouth. Remove all nearby objects that may pose a danger to the patient. Try to prevent injury by easing a falling patient to the floor and by cushioning the patient's head with a pillow, towel, or other soft material.

STROKE

A stroke or cerebrovascular accident (CVA) results in a loss of brain function. The two major causes are intracranial hemorrhage (hemorrhagic stroke) and loss of blood supply due to an embolus or other cause (ischemic stroke). Approximately 500,000 strokes occur each year in the United States with about 30% resulting in death. It is not necessary to differentiate the cause of a stroke in determining a course of action in dealing with a patient who may be having one. The case history is of some help here in identifying patients with either a history of stroke or a predisposition to stroke such as hypertension or atherosclerosis.

Signs and symptoms of stroke depend directly on the area of the brain that is affected, the seriousness of a CVA, and the severity. Some common signs and symptoms are listed in Table 7–1. It should be noted that none of these symptoms alone are unique to stroke.

The patient exhibiting signs or symptoms of a stroke should be placed in a comfortable position. If unconscious, the patient should be placed in a supine position. *EMS should be summoned immediately.* Until EMS arrives, the optometrist should monitor the ABCs and provide basic life support if breathing should stop.

Table 7–1   Signs and Symptoms of Stroke

Headache
Dizziness
Nausea and vomiting
Vertigo
Drowsiness
Weakness in arm or leg
Defects in speech
Unconsciousness

DIABETIC EMERGENCIES

Diabetes is on the rise in the United States. From 1990 to 1999, there was nearly a 40% increase in the number of diabetics. If this trend continues, more than 10% of the U.S. population will have diabetes in less than 10 years. There are two types of diabetic emergencies, hyperglycemia (increased blood sugar) and hypoglycemia (low blood sugar, or insulin shock). It is not practical or necessary for the optometrist to differentiate the two types as the treatment is the same for both.

The optometric record should contain detailed information about patients who are diabetic as well as an alert or warning on the patient's file. This alerts the examiner that certain signs and symptoms may be the result of a diabetic emergency. Knowing that the patient is diabetic is the best clue to recognizing a diabetic emergency. The most common signs and symptoms are presented in Table 7–2. However, one should not depend on "classic" symptoms. If a diabetic patient exhibits any abnormal signs or symptoms, suspect a diabetic emergency.

First aid for either hyperglycemia or hypoglycemia is the same. If the patient is conscious, *give sugar and call EMS.* The sugar will help in hypoglycemia and will not harm the patient with hyperglycemia. This is the case primarily because the onset of hypoglycemia is rapid and the onset of hyperglycemia may occur over several days. The best form for the administration of sugar is sugar dissolved in water, hard candy, or orange juice sipped slowly.

Table 7–2 Signs and Symptoms of Diabetic Emergencies

Hyperglycemia
   Thirst
   Frequent urination
   Fatigue
   Headache
   Shortness of breath
   Blurred vision
   Nausea and vomiting
   Red, hot, dry skin
   Sweet or fruity (acetone) breath
   Mental stupor
Hypoglycemia
   Has not eaten for several hours
   Diminished cerebral function
   Lethargy
   Cold, wet skin
   May appear intoxicated

ANAPHYLAXIS (ANAPHYLACTIC SHOCK)

Anaphylaxis is a severe, life-threatening, allergic reaction to an allergen such as a drug, food, or insect sting, to which the patient has been previously sensitized. Many patients know of their allergies and will report them in the case history. Some will not. Since the onset of an anaphylactic reaction is rapid (1 to 15 minutes), it rarely occurs in the optometric office except as a reaction to a drug that is being administered.

An anaphylactic reaction is extremely serious because it can cause:

- laryngeal swelling
- bronchial constriction
- edema of the epiglottis and larynx

All of the above contribute to an obstructed airway leading to a breathing emergency. If no action is taken, death can occur within minutes.

The practitioner should be aware of the most common life-threatening signs and symptoms of anaphylaxis (Table 7–3).

The most important thing the optometrist can do for a patient in anaphylactic shock is to *call EMS immediately*. While awaiting EMS, it is essential to keep the airway open and to institute rescue breathing if breathing stops. It may also be necessary to start CPR and/or defibrillate if the patient's heart stops (see Chapter 8).

If available, the following adjunct therapy is advised while waiting for EMS:

1. Epinephrine (0.3–0.5 mL) administered parenterally. Patients who have a history of severe allergy often carry a kit containing a preloaded syringe or ampule and, if conscious, may inject the drug themselves.
2. Diphenhydramine (Benadryl)—25–50 mg orally or parenterally.
3. Oxygen.

Table 7–3 Signs and Symptoms of Life-Threatening Anaphylaxis

Tachycardia
Decreased blood pressure
Bronchospasm
Shock (decreased blood to vital organs)
Convulsions
Unconsciousness
Cardiovascular collapse

Chapter 8

Chest Pain

The most important distinction that must be made with chest pain is that between angina pectoris and acute myocardial infarction (also called AMI or heart attack). Heart attacks have a relatively high mortality within a very short time of the attack. Angina, while less serious, can be a precursor to a heart attack. There are other causes of chest pain but none are life-threatening. In hyperventilation, for example, there may be chest pain but the major symptom is shortness of breath and this breathing emergency can be dealt with effectively (see Chapter 6).

ANGINA PECTORIS

Angina pectoris may be defined as substernal chest pain or discomfort that is relieved by rest and/or the administration of nitroglycerin. It is not necessarily life-threatening. However, if the pain lasts for more than 15 minutes, it should be considered an acute myocardial infarction (AMI) or heart attack. The optometrist should be aware of prior history of heart problems (angina or AMI) via the case history. As much as possible, the optometrist should seek to have such patients relaxed, as stress can be a precipitating factor in angina pectoris.

Signs and symptoms of angina pectoris may be found in Table 8–1. It is important to remember that these could also be signs and symptoms of AMI.

First aid treatment for angina pectoris consists in having the patient rest in an upright position and, if available, the sublingual administration of nitroglycerin. Patients with a history of angina pectoris often have nitroglycerin tablets with them. The steps to take in caring for a patient with angina pectoris are presented in Table 8–2.

If the patient has no history of angina pectoris and, therefore, does not carry nitroglycerin, it is best to call EMS immediately. Administration of oxygen is helpful with angina patients as oxygen helps to keep the coronary ar-

Table 8-1   Signs and Symptoms of Angina Pectoris

Dull, aching substernal discomfort
Suffocating, heavy, or squeezing sensation
Pain radiating to arms, jaw, or scapular area
Nausea and vomiting
Shortness of breath
Anxiety

teries open. Oxygen can be administered in the absence of nitroglycerin or as an adjunct to nitroglycerin. If nitroglycerin and/or oxygen does not relieve the chest pain in a patient with no prior history of angina, EMS should be called within three to four minutes of the onset of chest pain.

ACUTE MYOCARDIAL INFARCTION (AMI)

A heart attack (AMI, or acute myocardial infarction) is, unfortunately, a quite common occurrence in the United States (over 1 million cases per year) and nearly half are fatal. They can occur in women as well as men. Children and infants rarely suffer heart attacks except as the result of breathing emergencies.

The most common symptom of a heart attack is chest pain. It may be severe or relatively mild. However, any chest pain in a patient *with a prior history* of chest pain that is not relieved by relaxation or nitroglycerin within 10 to 15 minutes should be managed as a potential AMI. *Without a prior history*, the patient should be managed as a potential AMI within three to four minutes of the onset of chest pain. The signs and symptoms of a heart attack are listed in Table 8-3. It is far better to recognize symptoms early and to get the patient into the hands of advanced medical care personnel than it is to deal with a heart that has stopped beating.

Treatment of an AMI requires *prompt* management and calling EMS promptly. In cases of cardiac arrest, early CPR, early defibrillation, and ad-

Table 8-2   Management of Angina Pectoris in Patient with Prior History of Chest Pain

Position patient in upright position
Calm the patient
Administer nitroglycerin: 1 tab q5min up to 3 times
If pain does not subside, call EMS
Monitor the ABCs and provide basic life support as necessary

Table 8–3 Signs and Symptoms of a Heart Attack

Pain—pressing or crushing sensation
Lasts longer than angina pain (>15 min)
Cold sweat
Apprehension—fear of "impending doom"
Shortness of breath
Levine's sign—hand clutching at chest

vanced cardiac life support are essential elements of care. Therefore, recognizing the signs and symptoms of a heart attack and taking *prompt* action are crucial. Seconds count! The management is essentially the same as for angina pectoris. Once EMS has been summoned, it is extremely important to monitor the patient's ABCs and vital signs. Should the patient go into cardiac arrest during the optometric examination, the examiner should be prepared to perform CPR and, if available, to provide early automated defibrillation.

Patient Has No Pulse

In checking the patient, it has been determined that:

The patient is unconscious
The patient is not breathing
The patient has no pulse

After the patient has been checked and EMS has been summoned, cardiopulmonary resuscitation (CPR) should be started as quickly as possible in order to circulate oxygenated blood to the brain. It is not likely that CPR will restart the heart, but automated external defibrillation (AED) may.

CPR is performed using a combination of chest compressions (Figure 8–1) and breaths (Figure 8–2). The ratio is 15 compressions to two breaths for an adult and five compressions to one breath for a child or infant. The carotid pulse should be rechecked after the first minute and every few minutes after that. If the patient has a pulse, but is not breathing, rescue breathing should be administered. Again, it is strongly recommended that optometrists take a course in CPR and become certified to perform the procedure.

Once begun, CPR should continue until:

1. EMS personnel arrive and take over, or
2. another rescuer arrives and takes over, or

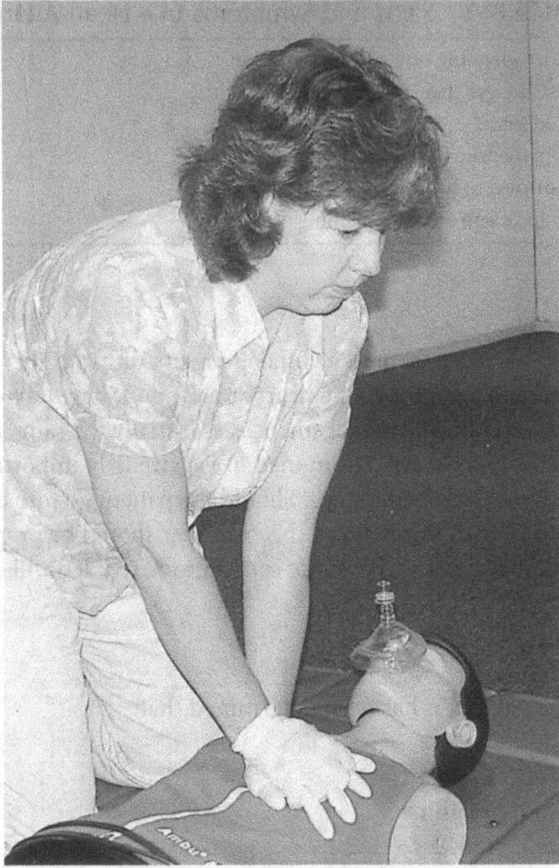

Figure 8–1. Giving chest compressions during CPR.

3. the victim regains pulse (continue with rescue breathing if still not breathing), or
4. the rescuer is too exhausted to continue, or
5. an automated defibrillator becomes available.

Use of an Automated External Defibrillator (AED)

An AED is a machine that analyzes the heart's rhythm and, if necessary, tells the rescuer to deliver a shock to a victim of sudden cardiac arrest. This shock may help the heart to reestablish an effective rhythm. The AED requires no decision, on the part of the rescuer, as to whether or not to deliver a shock. There are, however, a number of precautions that one must take in using an AED.

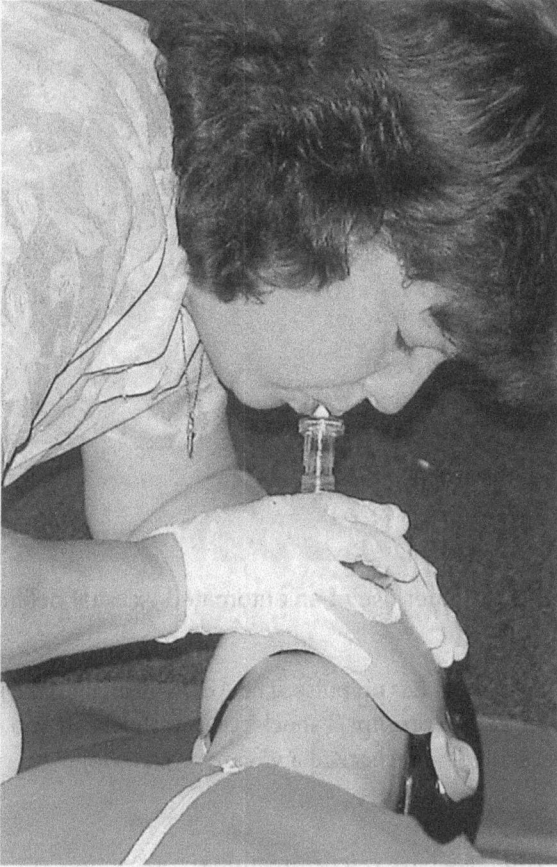

Figure 8–2. Giving breaths during CPR.

Therefore, it is essential that the user of an AED be properly trained. AED training is now commonly given as part of CPR training. An illustration of a commonly used AED is shown in Figure 8–3.

The AED is rapidly becoming the standard of care for first aid in cases of cardiac arrest. These machines can be found in many public places including airports, airplanes, restaurants, shopping malls, and in most health facilities. First responders to emergencies, including many police vehicles, are now equipped with AEDs. The AED is not to be confused with the more complex defibrillators used in hospitals or by paramedics. These require judgment as to when to deliver a shock and what the strength of the shock should be. More information on AED machines is presented in Chapter 9.

If an AED is immediately available, it should be utilized as soon as it is de-

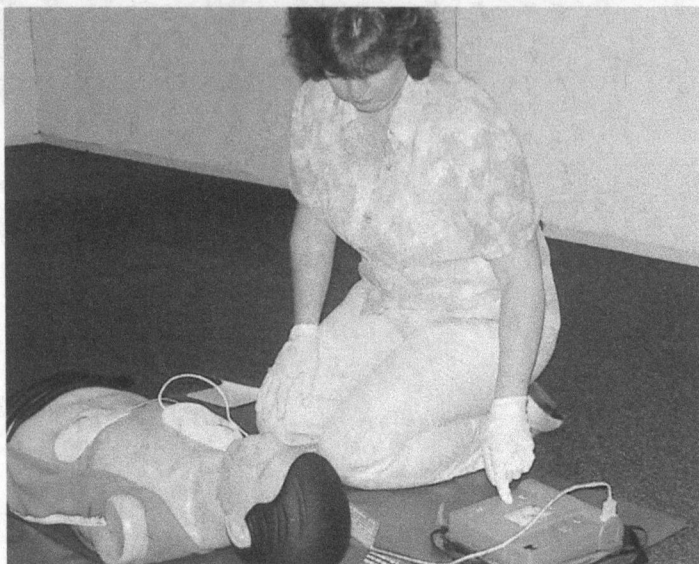

Figure 8–3. Proper use of an automated external defibrillator.

termined that the patient has no pulse. The AED will analyze the heart rhythm and advise (with a voice prompt) "shock" or "no shock." If "no shock" is advised, the pulse should be rechecked and care given as follows:

No pulse—Give CPR
Pulse but no breathing—Give rescue breathing
Breathing and has a pulse—Monitor the ABCs

The AED remains attached to the patient and keeps reanalyzing the heart rhythm. If CPR is resumed, it is possible that the AED will, at some point, advise another shock.

  If CPR has been started and is in progress, and an AED becomes available, the rescuer can prepare to use the AED immediately after a pulse check (assuming that the patient has no pulse).

  The use of an AED is a situation where it is better to have two trained rescuers available. Therefore, it is wise for office staff to be trained in emergency care procedures. Training of office staff is discussed in Chapter 9.

Being Prepared

Once everything that can be done to prevent an emergency has been done, the next best thing is to be prepared to deal with life-threatening emergencies. Since the optometrist has a responsibility to his or her patient to respond if that patient experiences a life-threatening emergency in the optometric setting, it is the optometrist who should take the lead in making sure that appropriate equipment and training are available.

OFFICE PROCEDURES

Depending upon the setting, various office procedures such as clinical care protocols, billing, and personnel policy are more or less formalized. In many instances, there are very specific procedures spelled out in writing and incorporated into a manual. Procedures for dealing with life-threatening emergencies should be part of any such manual and should be carefully spelled out for all office personnel. These procedures should be prominently posted so that they are available immediately to all office personnel. There are several essential elements (Table 9–1).

Code for Responding

It may be quite upsetting for patients in the reception area, as well as the family of a patient experiencing a life-threatening emergency, for the optometrist to be shouting "help" or "emergency" or a similar unsettling phrase. Having a preset emergency code such as "code blue" or some other appropriate phrase to communicate that an emergency is occurring would be preferable. It is important that whoever witnesses the emergency calls for the help of another office staff person either to assist in the care of the patient or to be available to call EMS. The "code" can be shouted, phoned on an intercom, or, if available, called over a public address system as is customary in hospitals.

Table 9–1 Essential Elements of Office Procedure for Dealing with Life-Threatening Emergencies

Code for responding
Emergency phone numbers
Location of emergency supplies/equipment
Step-by-step procedures for applying emergency care skills (CPR, AED, etc.)

Emergency Phone Numbers

The most important phone number is that of the local EMS provider (see Chapter 5, section on calling EMS). Other phone numbers that may be helpful to have include a consulting physician, the local poison control center, and the emergency room of the local hospital. As part of the patient's clinical record, there should be an emergency contact number for that patient so that a relative or friend can be notified, as well as the phone number of the patient's primary care physician.

Location of Emergency Supplies/Equipment

The office procedures should state specifically where supplies and equipment are kept so that minimal time is lost in getting the needed supplies and equipment to the patient. Preferably, a staff person will bring these to the person who is caring for the patient. Such supplies and equipment might include:

First aid kit
Disposable gloves
Breathing devices
Automated external defibrillator
Oxygen

The procedures should also assign responsibility for maintaining emergency supplies and equipment. An AED, for example, requires that the battery be checked regularly. Medications in the first aid kit need to be checked for expiration dates. First aid kits may need to be restocked.

Step-by-Step Procedures

Even when office personnel have taken training courses in dealing with emergencies, it is sometimes difficult to remember exactly what to do when an ac-

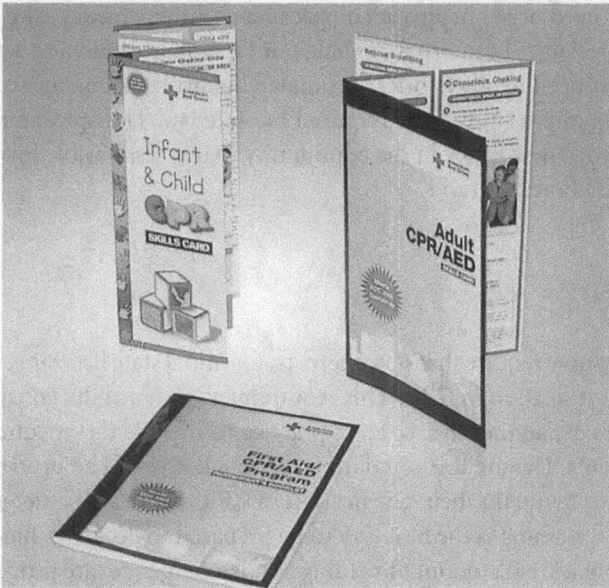

Figure 9–1. Skills card and participant manual (American Red Cross).

tual emergency occurs. Supplemental materials that deal with specific procedures and skills can be helpful. The materials can be prepared by office staff or purchased from a variety of sources.

The American Red Cross, for example, utilizes a series of "skills cards" in its training courses, which make excellent references for such procedures as checking the patient, rescue breathing, CPR, and the use of an AED. These skills cards make for excellent references in an emergency (Figure 9–1).

At the high-cost end there are devices available that provide an audio voice to guide the rescuer through various scenarios. A scenario is invoked by pressing a button on the device such as: "unconscious," "no pulse," or "not breathing."

There is, however, no substitute for appropriate training and regular practicing of the procedures involved in responding to an emergency.

CONSULTING PHYSICIAN

While it is not required as part of an emergency procedure, it is highly desirable for the optometrist to develop a relationship with a physician who can advise on office emergency procedures and who would be available by phone should the need arise. A physician specializing in emergency care would be ideal but specialists in internal medicine or cardiology could also serve in this role. If the office intends to offer automated defibrillation, an agreement with a consulting physician may be required by state law. The optometrist should check this with the agency in the community that is responsible for public access defibrillation programs.

TRAINING

Many states now require that optometrists, for initial state licensing, must have a current certification in CPR. This requirement was introduced with the advent of laws expanding the scope of practice to include therapeutic pharmaceutical agents. Having this standard established, it would be prudent for optometrists to maintain their certification in CPR and related emergency care. Such formal training is the best way to be prepared to deal with life-threatening emergencies. No amount of reading about emergency care procedures can substitute for the practical nature of emergency care training.

Excellent training is available through the American Heart Association or the American Red Cross either directly or through a third party such as a hospital, community agency, college or school, or a commercial provider. Such courses are also beginning to be offered as part of optometric continuing education programs. A good starting point to finding an appropriate course would be the local chapter of the American Heart Association or American Red Cross.

There are several levels of course offerings. Most courses are offered for the lay person and require little or no medical or technical background. One should begin with a basic-level course in CPR and, if possible, one including training in automated defibrillation. Such a course is perfectly adequate but individuals may wish to continue with courses leading to certification in basic life support or even advanced life support. Special short courses are also available in such areas as oxygen administration and the use of various breathing devices. Separate courses are offered for dealing with children and infants and these should be considered for offices where significant numbers of children and infants are seen.

It is definitely advantageous for office personnel, other than optometrists, to be trained. Procedures such as AED and two-person CPR are often more effective than one-rescuer techniques. In addition, having more than one person who knows what to do in an emergency is a significant advantage in providing effective and timely care to a patient experiencing a life-threatening emergency.

UNIVERSAL PRECAUTIONS

There are very few reported cases of rescuers, in emergency situations, contracting diseases from victims that they have helped. It is recommended, however, that basic infection control procedures be followed in dealing with patients who are experiencing a life-threatening emergency, particularly if rescue breathing or another procedure requiring mouth-to-mouth contact is necessary. While various breathing devices are available (see below), none are guaranteed to totally remove the possibility of bacterial or viral transmission. Likewise, direct contact with bodily fluids should be avoided.

The most important element in infection control is the use of disposable gloves. These gloves should be readily available in the examination room. In addition, they should be included within the office's first aid kit. It would be helpful to have different sizes available as well as nonlatex gloves for those individuals who may have an allergy to latex. Caution should be exercised in removing disposable gloves so that the external surfaces do not come into direct contact with the rescuer's skin (Figure 9–2).

Proper receptacles for contaminated medical waste should be available for the disposal of gloves, gauze, or any other material that may have been in contact with body fluids. Used needles and syringes should be placed in a container approved for this purpose.

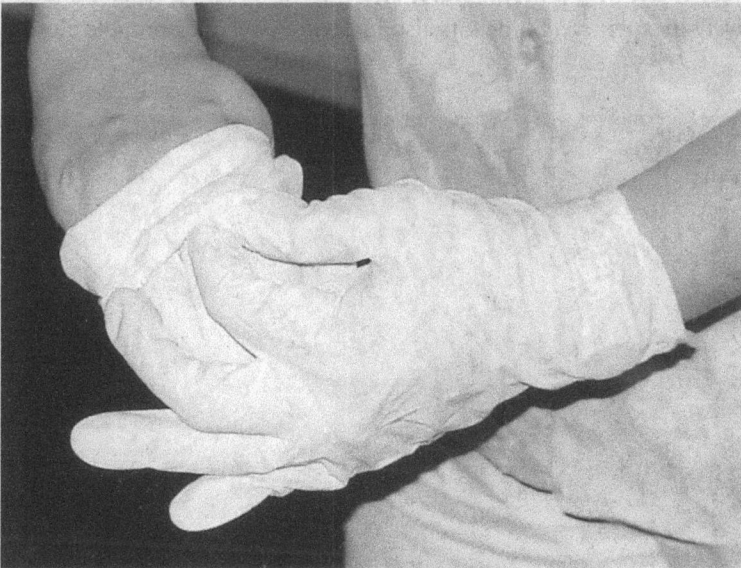

Figure 9–2. Proper removal of disposable gloves.

BREATHING DEVICES

There are a number of relatively inexpensive devices available that alleviate the need for direct mouth-to-mouth contact when it is necessary to perform rescue breathing or CPR. The devices enable the rescuer to achieve an effective seal over the patient's nose and mouth and to deliver breaths. Many of the devices are equipped with either filters or one-way valves that help to prevent air and microorganisms from passing from the patient to the rescuer. None, however, are absolutely guaranteed to prevent disease transmission.

Face Shields

A variety of face shields (Figure 9–3) are readily available and easy to carry. They range from shields carried in a key chain device to those with inserts that go into the patient's mouth. Shields are normally used in training courses and may be convenient as a device to carry in pocket or purse but they are not as effective as the other devices described below that should be considered for in-office use.

Face Mask

A commonly available pocket face mask kit (Figure 9–4), which is comprised of a face mask with a mouthpiece, one-way valve, and a replaceable filter, is relatively inexpensive. Some kits also include a pair of disposable gloves.

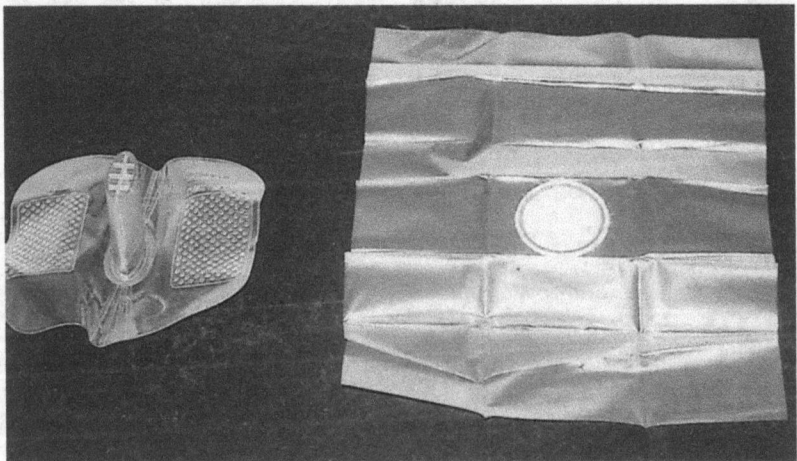

Figure 9–3. Commonly used face shields.

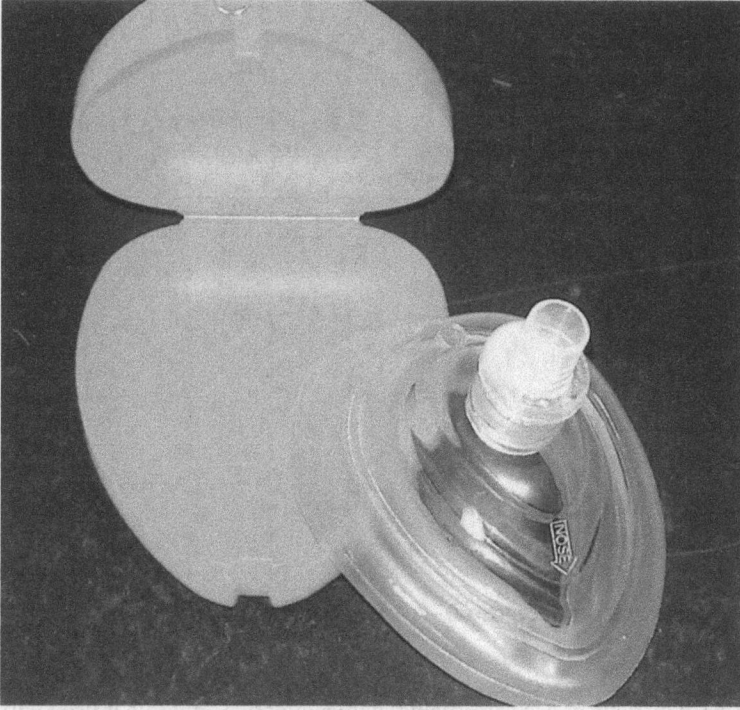

Figure 9–4. Pocket face mask.

Bag-Valve Mask

This device (Figure 9–5) consists of a face mask attached to a large plastic bulb that is squeezed by the rescuer to "breathe" atmospheric air into the victim. This device has several advantages over those described previously. The air being delivered is atmospheric air, which contains about 21% oxygen, as opposed to exhaled air, which contains about 16% oxygen. There is no risk of disease transmission either from patient to rescuer or from rescuer to patient. The device can accommodate a supplementary oxygen supply.

There is one disadvantage of this device in that it usually requires two people to use it properly and effectively. One person keeps the face mask portion in place while the other delivers the air.

AUTOMATED DEFIBRILLATORS

As with any new technology, improved automated external defibrillators (AEDs) are coming onto the market frequently and prices are decreasing (Fig-

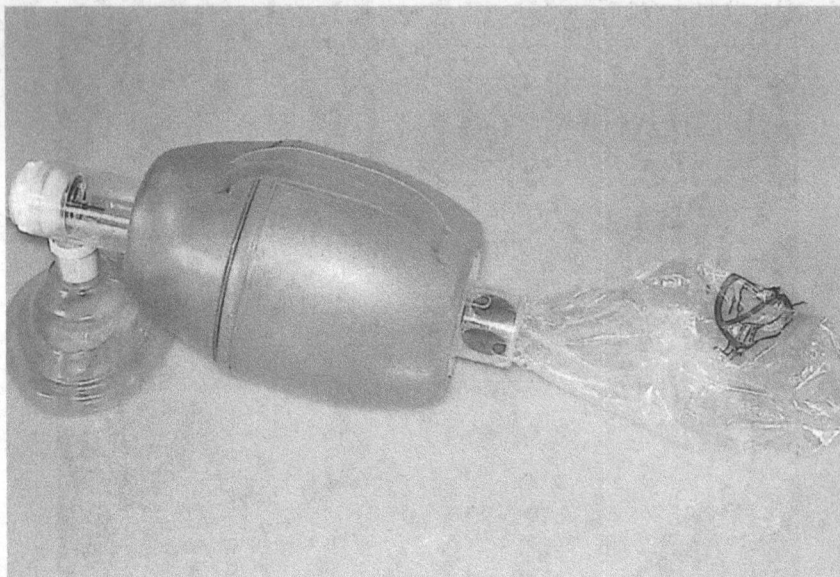

Figure 9–5. Bag-valve mask.

ure 9–6). The devices are extremely reliable, effective, and safe if used with the precautions taught in training courses. The technique for using AEDs is relatively uncomplicated but it must be taught as part of a complete CPR course.

The AED should be placed in a location where it is easily accessible both for use and for monitoring the battery charge. The devices use lithium batteries as a power source to deliver shocks to the patient and these must be replaced when indicated.

The devices are available from most medical supply companies, through the American Red Cross or American Heart Association, or directly from any one of several manufacturers. The most commonly used devices in the United States are those manufactured by Hewlett-Packard Corporation, Survivalink Corporation, and Medtronic Corporation.

FIRST AID KIT

In addition to equipment and supplies for dealing with ocular emergencies, it is important to have readily available those items of equipment and supplies most likely to be needed to deal with medical emergencies. Unlike ocular emergencies, where the optometrist is likely to want to be as fully equipped as possible, medical emergencies call only for those supplies necessary for first

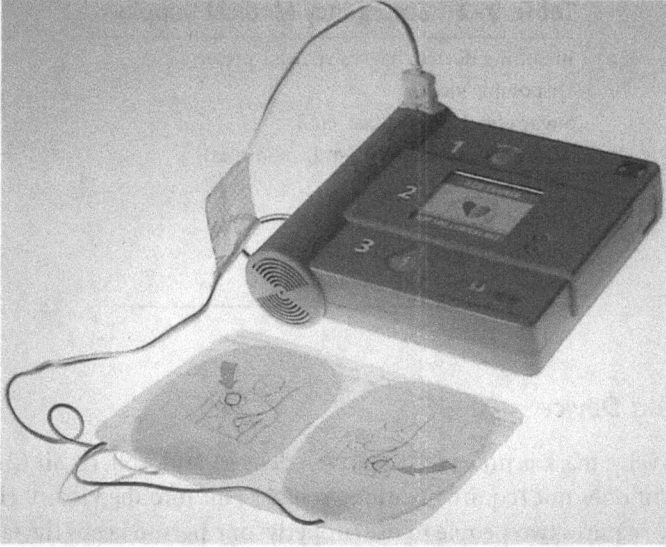

Figure 9–6. An automated external defibrillator (AED).

aid response to life-threatening emergencies. It is not necessary to create a miniature hospital emergency room.

It is important to bear in mind that no first aid kit is a substitute for the optometrist, and other personnel, being trained in how to deal with medical emergencies. Simply having the proper first aid supplies and equipment is not enough. There is no substitute for being prepared in emergency care skills through training courses and for practicing how to deal with emergencies by having regular drills involving all office staff.

A standard first aid kit equipped to deal with many non-life-threatening emergencies should be available in the office. These kits may be purchased commercially or they may be assembled from items readily available from the local pharmacy. First aid kits usually contain various types of wound dressings, antiseptics, a triangular bandage for a sling, a cold pack, and implements such as scissors and tweezers. They may also contain items for protection of the rescuer such as disposable gloves and breathing barriers. In addition to the standard items, it is necessary to have the additional supplies and equipment needed to deal with life-threatening emergencies.

A list of suggested items for an expanded first aid kit is provided in Table 9–2. This is not a complete list of items in that what is included in the first aid kit in any office represents the personal choice of the optometrist as well as what is required and/or allowable under applicable state law. For example, in certain states, optometrists are specifically permitted to use injectable drugs.

Table 9-2 Emergency Medical Supplies

Breathing device (bag-valve mask preferred)
Disposable gloves
Sugar (candy, fruit juice, etc.)
Aromatic ammonia (0.3-mL vaporoles)
Inhaler (bronchodilator)
Nitroglycerin tablets or spray
Diazepam (oral, 10-15 mg.)
Epinephrine (1-mL ampules)

Breathing Device

The bag-valve mask is preferred because it delivers atmospheric air (21% oxygen) and it does not require breathing rescuer's air into the victim. However, it usually requires two people to use properly; one person keeps the face mask in place while the other delivers the air. The pocket face mask (Figure 9-4) with filter is a perfectly acceptable alternative.

Disposable Gloves

These should be of the hypoallergenic variety and kept with the first aid supplies. Pairs of different sizes (small, medium, and large) would be desirable.

Sugar

Sugar, in almost any readily available form (candy, fruit juice, cane sugar solution), is necessary for the management of diabetic emergencies (hypoglycemia or hyperglycemia).

Aromatic Ammonia

Supplied as vaporoles or ampules or as a solution of aromatic spirts of ammonia, this is often a quite effective remedy for patients who have fainted and should be a part of any first aid kit.

Inhaler

Asthmatics will most likely have their own but having one available in the office is still a good idea.

Nitroglycerin

Nitroglycerin is available in tablet or spray form. The dosage is from 0.3 mg to 0.6 mg. Tablets are administered sublingually, one every five minutes up to three tablets; then call EMS if there is no relief. One or two metered sprays are recommended with no more than three sprays in 15 minutes. Patients with a history of chest pain will usually have their own medication with them and this is preferred as it will be their correct dosage. For patients with no prior history of chest pain, EMS should be summoned within two minutes.

Diazepam (Valium)

Diazepam (10–15 mg) is administered orally in cases of hyperventilation *only* if breathing into a paper bag does not work.

Epinephrine (Adrenaline)

In cases of severe allergic reaction (anaphylaxis), and if the optometrist has the legal authority, an injection of epinephrine is the treatment of choice. Often the patient with a known severe allergy has ampules of epinephrine and, if conscious, may inject him- or herself. Benadryl (25–50 mg) is also effective and can be administered in oral as well as injectable form.

Other forms of management are preferable to the use of drugs. Medications should only be used when these do not seem to be effective. In any case, where a patient experiencing a potentially life-threatening emergency does not respond to recommended management, EMS should be summoned immediately.

Chapter 10

Medical-Legal Considerations

This chapter does not purport to give specific legal advice. Rather, it addresses several concepts that relate to the optometrist providing emergency care in the patient care setting and in the course of daily life as a family member, friend, or passerby.

The overriding message is that, in the patient care setting, the optometrist has no choice. Emergency care must be provided to a patient who experiences a life-threatening emergency. With the passage of many of the diagnostic and therapeutic drug bills in various states, certification in cardiopulmonary resuscitation (CPR) became required either upon initial licensure or upon the expansion of the license to include either diagnostic or therapeutic drugs. Optometrists who are institutionally employed, such as in hospitals, schools of optometry, and other clinics, are usually required to have CPR certification as part of their credentialing for a staff position and they are expected to renew that certification as necessary.

In responding to a medical emergency, either in the optometric setting or on the outside, the optometrist is considered similar to a lay person who is trained in first aid (including CPR) or what is considered a "first responder" or "citizen responder" in most emergency medical systems. It is his or her responsibility to keep the patient alive until more highly trained personnel, such as an emergency medical technician, a paramedic or a physician trained in emergency care, arrive. Several key legal concepts (Table 10–1) are explained as follows:

DUTY TO ACT

As explained above, it is the optometrist's duty to act when he or she is serving as provider of care to the patient who experiences a life-threatening emergency in the optometric setting. This includes calling the local emergency medical services entity, performing lifesaving skills for which the optometrist

Table 10-1   Some Key Medical-Legal Concepts

Duty to act
Good Samaritan laws
Standard of care
Negligence
Abandonment
Confidentiality
Record keeping

should be currently certified, and having ready access to the necessary supplies and equipment required to do so. Outside of the optometric setting, however, the optometrist's duty to act is the same as a layperson's. He or she may choose to act or not to act. That choice may be based on a number of personal considerations and, while there may be a moral duty to act, there is no legal duty to act. At the very least, however, when confronted with a life-threatening emergency, the optometrist, or any other bystander, should call the emergency services number and report the incident.

GOOD SAMARITAN LAWS

Good Samaritan laws exist in every state. They were instituted to protect medical doctors who stop to help individuals in life-threatening situations such as serious injuries in an auto accident. In essence, any individual is covered by provisions of these laws if he or she renders appropriate care to an individual who is experiencing a medical emergency. It does not mean that one cannot be sued but it does offer some protection against liability in these circumstances. However, it is rare for lawsuits to be instituted against individuals who render assistance in emergency situations, regardless of the outcome.

STANDARD OF CARE

For the purposes of providing emergency care in the optometric setting, standard of care may defined as "doing what an ordinarily prudent optometrist would do in similar circumstances" or "not doing what an ordinarily prudent optometrist would not do in similar circumstances." It also means, for example, that, when providing CPR, it should be provided according to the standards for the CPR course in which the optometrist is certified. If you do not meet the standard of care and your actions harm another person, you may be successfully sued.

NEGLIGENCE

Negligence is failure to follow a reasonable standard of care, thereby causing injury or damage to another. Failure to recognize obvious signs of a medical emergency, giving improper treatment, or failing to summon EMS personnel could all be considered examples of negligence.

ABANDONMENT

Simply stated, abandonment means stopping emergency care once it has been instituted. You must not stop giving care unless

1. you are relieved by someone with an equal or higher level of training such as an EMT, paramedic, or emergency care physician, or
2. you are too exhausted to continue.

CONFIDENTIALITY

In the optometric setting, any information with regard to the patient's medical emergency is treated with the same confidentiality as for other parts of the patient's record. Outside of the optometric setting, similar confidentiality should be maintained and information not divulged to anyone except emergency medical services personnel or police.

RECORD KEEPING

It is important that a careful written record of the incident be created as soon as possible afterward, even if that turns out to be hours later.

Part II

OCULAR URGENCIES AND EMERGENCIES

Chapter 11

Ocular Foreign Bodies

"Doctor, I felt something go into my eye."

SCOPE OF THE PROBLEM

Ocular foreign bodies account for a significant number of injuries to the eye and have the potential to create severe structural damage and loss of vision. Depending on the nature of the injury, immediate intervention may be necessary in order to preserve sight. Some foreign bodies can be managed relatively easily in the office while others require immediate referral. A wide variety of ocular foreign bodies have been reported, the most common being metallic. Others include gunshot injuries and remnants from explosions. Rapid assessment including mechanism of injury, localization of the object, and evaluation of tissue damage is crucial in developing an appropriate plan of action.

HISTORY

Patients typically seek immediate attention following ocular foreign body injury. The vast majority of these patients are male. It is not uncommon for them to present with intense pain, reduced vision, injection, chemosis, and photophobia. Such patients are apt to present to the hospital emergency room as well as the practitioner's office. Individuals suffering from lesser injuries may complain of a sandy, gritty feeling or that "something is in the eye."

Alternatively, in cases of superficial injuries, the patient may not be aware that a foreign body is lodged in the eye. A projectile object may enter the eye at very high speed, cause a minimal entrance wound, and not initially produce pain. Orbital inflammation and pain on eye movements have been reported months after penetration by an intraorbital foreign body. The clinician should investigate any instances of periocular trauma to rule out the presence of a foreign body.

Table 11–1 Sources of Ocular Foreign Bodies

More common

Hammering on metal, with or without a chisel
Gunshot/BB gun
Industrial accidents
Gardening accidents
Children's accidents while playing

Less common

Hammering on concrete
Explosions
Traffic accidents

Ask about circumstances surrounding the injury.

History involves determining the circumstances surrounding the injury, the onset of injury, and the composition, size, and entry force of the foreign body. Metal striking metal is the most common cause of ocular foreign bodies. Thus it is important for the doctor to inquire as to whether the patient has been involved in any hammering, chiseling, or use of grinding machinery (Table 11–1).

The particular substance of the foreign body influences the amount of ocular damage, urgency of action, prognosis, and method of extraction. Every effort should be made to determine the composition of the material. In cases where location of the object is not obvious, the object becomes easier to find if the examiner is aware of what he or she is looking for. If possible, a piece of material should be brought into the examination for evaluation.

Determine the composition of the foreign body.

Foreign body substances may be divided into *organic, inorganic metallic,* and *inorganic nonmetallic* (Table 11–2). Organic foreign bodies such as wood and vegetable matter are associated with a high risk of inflammation and infection such as endophthalmitis (Table 11–3). Inorganic materials vary as to the extent to which they induce ocular inflammation. Some metallic materials, including copper, iron, and iron-containing substances like steel, are apt to cause severe ocular inflammation, while others, such as gold, silver, aluminum, and nickel, produce milder reactions. Common sources of injury, BB pellets are composed mostly of lead, with some iron.

Organic and some metallic materials are associated with increased risk of inflammation.

Relatively inert inorganic, nonmetallic substances, such as rubber, plastic,

Table 11–2 Ocular Foreign Body Substances

Organic

Wood

Vegetable matter

Cilia

Inorganic Nonmetallic

Rubber

Glass

Plastic

Stone

Inorganic Metallic

Copper

Iron

Steel

Lead

Aluminum

Nickel

Gold

Silver

BB pellets (lead + iron)

glass, and stone, tend to produce less inflammation, as do cilia. It is important to bear in mind that a relatively benign substance may be contaminated with noxious material that may render it harmful.

The clinician should attempt to determine the size of the penetrating object. Increased size of penetrating object is usually correlated with increased

Ask patient what actions were taken upon injury, when the last tetanus prophylaxis was, and whether safety glasses were worn.

Table 11–3 Severity of Inflammation Caused by Ocular Foreign Bodies

High	Medium	Low
Organic materials	Gold	Cilia
Copper	Silver	Rubber
Iron	Aluminum	Glass
Steel	Nickel	Plastic
		Stone

ocular damage. The actions taken by the patient should be investigated. For example, did the patient irrigate or manipulate the eye? Were any eyedrops used? It is also important to determine the date of the patient's last tetanus prophylaxis.

The clinician should also ask if the patient was wearing safety lenses at the time of the injury. Conventional lenses are often inadequate to protect patients from foreign body injury. The great majority of people with ocular foreign bodies were not wearing any eyewear at the time of injury, and even fewer were wearing safety eyewear.

Ocular history questions pertinent to any problem should not be omitted. Ocular symptomotology, such as pain, reduction in visual function, photophobia, and injection should be discussed. Can the patient localize the source of the pain? Are there any flashes or floaters, indicating a potential retinal tear or detachment? Is there diplopia, which may indicate an extraocular muscle restriction?

Ask about ocular symptoms.

Onset is crucial to determine, as time is frequently of the essence in managing ocular foreign bodies. Intervention often needs to be made within the first 24 hours in the event of penetrating injuries for the best outcome.

Primary Actions—History of a Patient with a Foreign Body

- Determine the onset of the injury
- Determine the substance of the foreign body
- Determine the circumstances regarding the injury
- Determine the nature and scope of the patient's symptoms

EXAMINATION

Classification of foreign bodies is based upon the location in which they are lodged: *superficial*, involving the conjunctiva or cornea, *intraocular*, involving the globe, and *intraorbital*, involving the orbit. When a patient suspected of having a foreign body is examined, an entire ocular health exam must be performed, including dilated fundus exam. Throughout the exam, minimal pressure should be placed on the globe in order to avoid further damage.

Perform a complete ocular health exam in patients with foreign bodies.

If the patient is unable to open the eye in order to take visual acuity, it may be necessary to insert a drop of topical anesthetic prior to taking visual acuity. Visual acuity will vary depending upon the extent of the injury and whether the visual axis is involved. A number of studies have shown that the initial visual acuity tends to be predictive of final visual acuity after the object is removed.

Take visual acuity. Anesthetic may be needed.

The suspected entry sight needs to be identified and investigated. When infection is suspected, the entry sight or piece of material that the foreign body came from should be cultured.

Identify and investigate the entry site. Determine if there is an open globe.

External exam should determine whether there is an open globe. This involves a full-thickness penetrating wound in the cornea or sclera. An open globe may occur in an entry wound from a previous surgery, such as cataract surgery. In the case of an eye presenting with extrusion of orbital contents, no further testing should be performed. An eye shield should be placed over the eye and the patient should immediately be referred for surgical repair.

If an open globe injury is suspected, a Seidel test should be performed. The suspected area of entry is painted with a moistened fluorescein strip. If under cobalt blue light the fluorescein turns black, there is evidence of a full-thickness wound and leakage of intraocular contents (Figure 11–1).

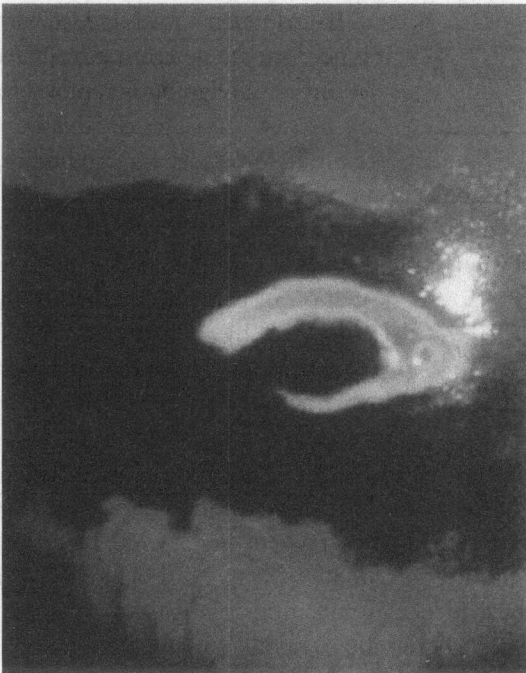

Figure 11–1. Positive Seidel sign indicating aqueous leak following trauma.

Assess EOMs and pupillary function.

Extraocular motility should be assessed to determine whether there is a limitation on movement. Foreign bodies may directly penetrate the extraocular muscles resulting in external ophthalmoplegia. Pupils should be assessed to evaluate for an afferent pupillary defect that may result from a foreign body penetrating the retina or optic nerve. Miosis may also be noted, which is often present in cases of acute anterior uveitis that may accompany foreign body injury.

Careful slit lamp exam should evaluate the lids, sclera, conjunctiva, and cornea for evidence of penetration. If a superficial foreign body is suspected,

Perform a careful slit lamp exam.

the upper lid should be double-everted to look for particles. This may be accomplished with the use of a Desmarres lid retractor. In examining the cornea and conjunctiva, the clinician should look for signs of conjunctival injection or chemosis,

particularly in the area of injury. In the cornea, common signs to be noted are linear epithelial fluorescein staining ("foreign body tracks"), superficial punctate keratitis, corneal edema, and corneal infiltrate. Metallic foreign bodies undergo siderosis (oxygenation) after 24 hours. An area of rust will be seen.

Determine the depth of a corneal foreign body.

If the foreign body is lodged within the cornea, it is necessary to determine what layer it is in. Regulations on foreign body removal by optometrists vary by state. In states in which optometrists are permitted to remove foreign bodies, removal may be prohibited if the object is posterior to the epithelium.

It should be noted that some superficial foreign bodies extract spontaneously without intervention. It is not uncommon for a patient to report the sensation of something entering the eye, the eye

Examine the anterior chamber, iris, and lens.

feeling scratchy and irritated, and no foreign body is found. However, there may be evidence of disturbance to the eye as revealed by conjunctival injection and corneal epithelial abrasion. In these

cases the patient may report that the symptoms have decreased. The anterior chamber should be examined for signs of cell or flare, which are often associated with ocular foreign bodies. Hypopyon, or white blood cells in the anterior chamber, indicates infection. Hyphema, or red blood cells in the anterior chamber, may be evidence of broken iris vessels.

The iris should be examined carefully for any presence of a foreign body, tear such as iridodialysis (disinsertion of the root of the iris from the ciliary body), or pupillary irregularity. Iris transillumination defects may indicate that the foreign body has penetrated the iris. Siderosis may result in areas of brown discoloration to the iris or lens. The anterior vitreous should be examined for cells. Endophthalmitis needs to be ruled out.

If intraocular penetration is suspected, gonioscopy needs to be performed to look for any penetration into the angle structures. This should not be performed if there is an open globe injury. Intraocular pressure (IOP) should be taken. A traumatic uveitis may result in an initial decrease in IOP. Penetrating injury will result in very low IOP.

Perform gonioscopy unless there is evidence of open globe.

Measure IOP.

All patients with ocular foreign bodies need to be dilated to examine the integrity of the posterior segment. In the case of a superficial foreign body in which no further ocular involvement is suspected, the clinician may examine the retina through an undilated pupil at the initial visit and defer dilation until the follow-up visit the next day. If posterior segment involvement is suspected, it is necessary to dilate the pupil at the first visit.

Perform a dilated fundus exam at some point in the care of the patient. Perform it immediately in cases of suspected intraocular foreign body.

Foreign bodies that have penetrated the vitreous may result in vitreous prolapse. Broken retinal blood vessels resulting from foreign body trauma may cause vitreal hemorrhage. The retina must be examined thoroughly to look for any abnormalities such as tears, holes, or detachment. Retinal inflammatory lesions may be signs of intraocular infection. Siderosis has the potential to cause retinal pigment epithelial degeneration. The electroretinogram (ERG) may become abnormal with time due to toxic metallosis. In cases of foreign bodies involving the retina, baseline ERG should be performed and repeated periodically, especially if the foreign body is left in place. The optic disc should be examined for any signs of hyperemia, elevation, or hemorrhage. If the foreign body results in traumatic optic neuropathy, pallor will not be seen at time of injury.

Order an ERG if a retinal foreign body is discovered.

In cases where an intraocular or intraorbital foreign body is suspected, imaging techniques such as plain X-ray films, CT scans, and MRIs may be employed in locating the foreign body. CT of the orbit with axial and coronal views is the standard. It is highly sensitive in identifying intraocular and intraorbital foreign bodies, with the ability to locate metallic objects as small as 0.5 mm in diameter.

Order imaging studies as needed. Remember the contraindications to MRI.

Table 11–4 Evaluation of Patients with Ocular Foreign Bodies

History

- Determine circumstances of injury
- Determine composition of foreign body
  - ○ If material is organic or is associated with severe inflammation, more immediate actions must be taken

Examination

- Complete ocular health exam
- Examine entry site
- Evaluate for possibility of open globe
  - ○ If open globe
    - Eye shield
    - Immediate referral
- Locate position of foreign body
  - ○ Perform CT scan
  - ○ If CT is negative, perform MRI, but only if object is known to be nonmetallic
  - ○ B-scan ultrasonography, ultrasound biomicroscopy used as adjunct

The use of the B-scan orbital ultrasound as well as a newer instrument, the ultrasound biomicroscope, may complement the CT scan in identifying the location and nature of the foreign body.

MRI provides the best resolution of soft tissue. However, because of its magnetic properties the use of an MRI can result in the movement of the foreign body. Therefore, it is contraindicated in the presence of magnetic and metallic foreign bodies. MRI is also contraindicated in individuals with cochlear implants, intracranial aneurysm clips, cardiac pacemakers, and defibrillators. CT is less effective at identifying wood, which is better imaged with MRI. If the CT fails to reveal the foreign body and a nonmetallic object is suspected, then an MRI is indicated (Table 11–4).

Primary Actions—Examination of a Patient with a Foreign Body

- Measure visual acuity, with prior use of topical anesthetic if necessary
- Identify and investigate the suspected entry sight
- Determine whether the globe is intact
- Perform complete ocular health exam to assess location of object and evaluate ocular tissues
- Perform imaging studies in cases in which intraorbital or intraocular foreign bodies are suspected

MANAGEMENT

In most cases, management of ocular foreign bodies involves extraction of the object with care taken to minimize tissue damage. Medical therapy is used for infection prophylaxis, to promote wound healing, or to enhance patient comfort. Secondary or tertiary care may be needed in cases of intraocular or intraorbital foreign bodies.

Superficial Foreign Bodies

Superficial conjunctival and corneal foreign bodies (Figure 11–2) are easily removed in the office setting. They often resolve with minimal or no scarring and without permanent reduction in visual acuity.

The eye is first anesthetized with topical drops such as proparacaine or tetracaine. The other eye may also be anesthetized to reduce reflexive blinking. Some very loosely embedded foreign bodies may be rinsed out of the eye with sterile saline or irrigating solution. The upper and lower lids

> *Very superficial foreign bodies may be removed with irrigation, a cotton-tipped applicator, or jeweler's forceps.*

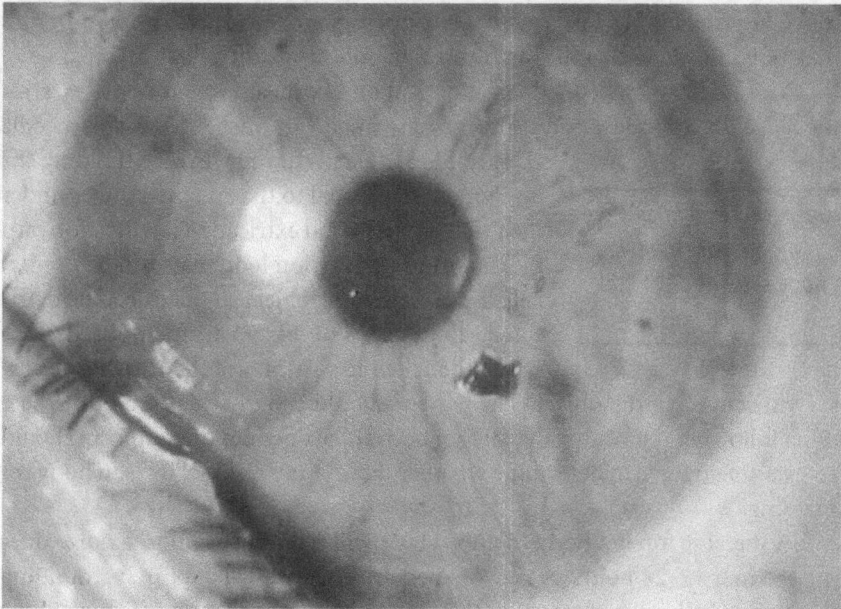

Figure 11–2. Metallic corneal foreign body.

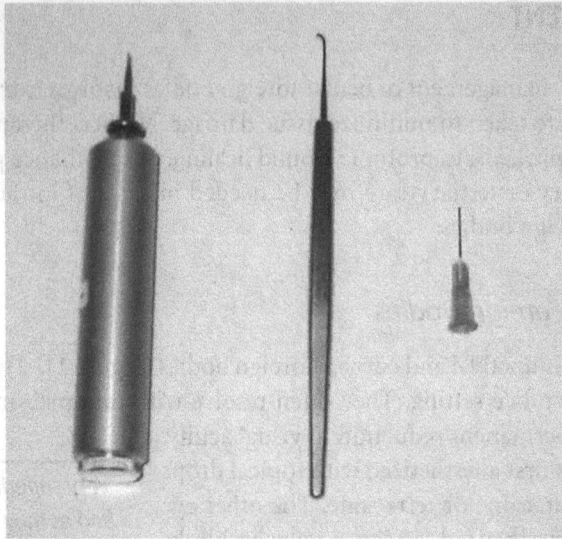

Figure 11–3. Equipment for foreign body removal.

should be everted to remove any remaining particles, which may be trapped in the conjunctival fornices. A moist cotton tip applicator may be used to remove any remaining loose particles. Superficial conjunctival foreign bodies may be removed with a moist cotton tip applicator or jeweler's forceps.

More deeply embedded conjunctival and corneal foreign bodies are removed with a foreign body spud or 25-gauge (5/8-inch) disposable needle (Figure 11–3). The technique involves holding the implement tangential to the eye, inserting it under the foreign object, and extricating it with a forward flicking motion. A nylon loop may also be used in helping to loosen the object so that it can be extricated. Regardless of the instrument used, care should be taken to disturb as little tissue as necessary in removing the object. The patient should experience some immediate relief following removal of the foreign body. If he does not, the clinician should re-examine the eye to determine whether there is any residual foreign body remaining.

Deeper foreign bodies are removed with a foreign body spud or disposable needle.

A metallic foreign body (Figure 11–2) will typically begin to oxidize during the first 12–24 hours. A ring-shaped area of rust will appear surrounding the object. Following removal of the foreign body, the rust ring (Figure 11–4) may be removed with a battery-operated ophthalmic drill such as an Alger brush. The instrument is spun manually to begin operation, then inserted tan-

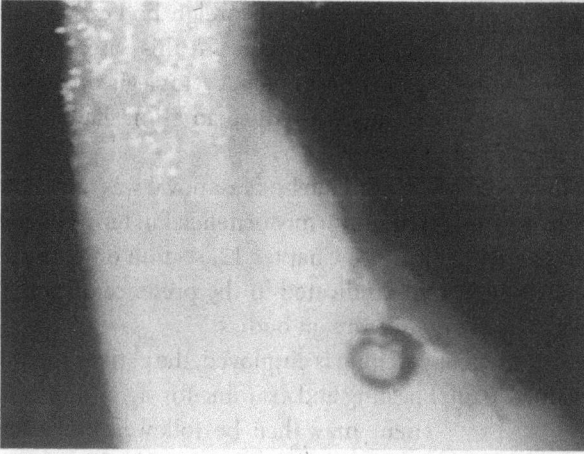

Figure 11–4. Corneal foreign body with rust ring.

gentially to the cornea as the area of rust is removed by making a divot in the cornea. The instrument will stop spinning if it meets too much resistance, thereby acting as a safety feature to prevent burrowing too deep into the cornea. The rust may alternatively be removed with a needle or spud. In the case of deeply embedded rust rings it is sometimes beneficial to delay removal for a day or two when the ring becomes more superficial as the epithelium begins to regenerate.

Use an Alger brush, needle, or spud to remove residual rust.

Some corneal foreign bodies are best not removed. Objects that are deeply embedded in the stroma, nontoxic, nonpainful, and close to the visual axis may be left in place if their extraction would result in disturbance of tissue significant enough to affect vision.

After removal of the foreign body, an epithelial abrasion will remain. The abrasion should be treated with broad-spectrum antibiotic prophylaxis. Well-tolerated antibiotic drops such as trimethoprim-polymyxin B q3h may be employed. Alternatively, ointments such as polysporin, bacitracin, or erythromycin may be used bid. Depending upon the degree of pain the patient is experiencing, nonsteroidal anti-inflammatory drops may also be used qid. These include ketorolac and diclofenac. Artificial tears may also be used for patient comfort. If the stroma is involved, a corneal scar will result.

After foreign body removal, use antibiotic prophylaxis and nonsteroidal anti-inflammatory agents for pain.

This scar has the potential to reduce vision by inducing irregular astigmatism.

Treat secondary uveitis with cycloplegia.

Superficial foreign bodies may also result in secondary uveitis. In this case, particularly if the patient is in pain, cycloplegic drops should be prescribed to reduce anterior chamber reaction and alleviate pain from ciliary spasm.

Patching the eye following foreign body removal was once common practice. It is no longer considered uniformly beneficial in terms of epithelial healing or reducing patient pain. (See Chapter 12, section on corneal abrasions.) In all cases, patching is contraindicated in the presence of potentially infectious materials such as organic foreign bodies.

Regardless of whether patching is employed, the patient should be seen the next day to evaluate ocular healing and examine for signs of infection. The patient may then be followed every few days, depending on the degree of healing, until the healing is complete. Eyedrops may be discontinued in a few days as well. As with the case of any abrasion, stromal edema (accompanied by reduction in visual acuity) may appear after removal of the foreign body. This typically resolves without treatment within a few days.

Examine the patient the day after foreign body removal.

Intraocular and Intraorbital Foreign Bodies

Intraocular (Figure 11–5) and intraorbital foreign bodies must be referred for ophthalmological evaluation. Immediate referral is important as inflammation and potential for infection increase with time. The patient should be advised to limit movement and be given an eye shield to be worn to prevent additional trauma. If the patient presents with a protruding foreign body, the case should be referred out for surgical removal. The object should not removed in the office.

Refer all cases of intraocular and intraorbital foreign body. Cover the eye with a shield before sending the patient to the consultant.

Patients with intraocular foreign bodies are hospitalized. Patients with intraorbital foreign bodies are usually hospitalized, though those not requiring surgical removal may be followed on an outpatient basis. The patient is started on antitetanus prophylaxis, if necessary. Broad-spectrum oral and intravenous antibiotics are employed immediately as prophylaxis for endophthalmitis.

Various surgical approaches are used for extraction, depending on the location of the foreign body and nature of the material. Most commonly,

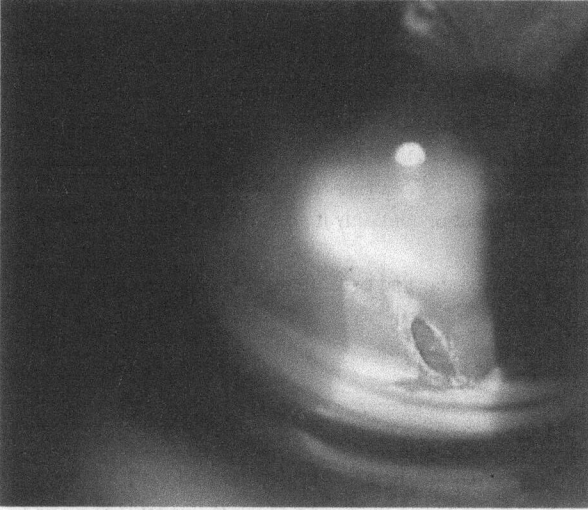

Figure 11–5. Intraocular foreign body.

intraocular foreign bodies are removed by pars plana vitrectomy through use of forceps. Surgical openings through the limbus may also be employed. In eyes containing magnetic foreign bodies, a magnet may be used to position the object to facilitate removal. In the case of intraorbital foreign bodies, transconjunctival, transseptal, or cranio-orbital entry ports have been used.

Inert foreign bodies, particularly those not threatening vision or those whose removal would cause substantial damage, are often left in place. If the foreign body is left in, the patient needs to be seen periodically to determine whether toxicity has developed. If the material is organic, or an inorganic material likely to cause significant inflammation, it is always removed.

Finally, patient education is critical. Many foreign body injuries can be prevented by use of safety goggles. Particularly when engaging in activities known to cause ocular foreign body injury such as hammering nails or grinding metal, the patient should be counseled to protect the eyes with safety materials (Table 11–5).

Primary Actions—Management of a Patient with a Foreign Body

- Remove superficial foreign bodies with implement of choice
- Remove any rust rings left by metallic objects with Alger brush or burr

Table 11–5   Management of Patients with Ocular Foreign Bodies

- Superficial
  - ○ Remove object with proper instrument
  - ○ Remove any rust ring
  - ○ Prescribe prophylactic antibiotic drops or ointment
  - ○ Prescribe cycloplegic in cases of uveitis or severe pain
  - ○ Patch with caution and only if necessary, never in cases of organic foreign bodies
  - ○ Follow up next day and thereafter until healing is complete
- Intraocular and intraorbital
  - ○ Prophylactic antibiotics
  - ○ Immediate referral

- Treat patient with antibiotics, NSAIDs, and cycloplegic agents
- Follow up the next day, and subsequently until the eye is healed
- Refer intraorbital or intraocular foreign bodies for evaluation for surgical extraction
- Educate patient on eye protection

Chapter 12

Ocular Trauma

"Doctor, I got hit in my eye and cannot see."

SCOPE OF THE PROBLEM

Trauma to the eye is one of the leading causes of visual impairment and blindness. Potentially devastating, ocular trauma carries with it not only the prospect of vision loss, but also the potential of facial disfigurement.

It is estimated that up to 2.4 million ocular injuries occur in the United States each year. One million of these entail permanent injury, of which 75% result in monocular blindness. Eye injury is second only to cataract as the most common cause of visual impairment.

Prevent Blindness America (formerly the National Society to Prevent Blindness) estimates that 90% of all ocular injuries are preventable. The United States Eye Injury Registry (USEIR), a federation of individual state eye injury registries formed in 1988, documents serious eye injuries (those judged to result in permanent structural or functional damage to the eye), collects epidemiological data, and disseminates information on the prevention and management of eye injuries to the public and eye care professionals (Table 12–1).

The majority of serious eye injuries occur to patients who are young and male. Males account for approximately 80% of those sustaining serious ocular injuries. Home is the most common place where injuries occur, with incidence on the increase. The workplace had been the most frequent place of injuries, but additional safety measures have resulted in their number declining. Motor vehicle crashes and highway accidents are also important sources of ocular injuries, as are sports and recreation.

Less than 15% of all serious ocular injuries are due to violence. However, the number can be as high as 43% in urban areas. Up to 34% of such incidents result in initial vision of no light perception (NLP). Sixteen percent of all ini-

Table 12–1 Characteristics of Ocular Injury

- Place of injury
  - ○ Home—40%
  - ○ Street/highway—13%
  - ○ Industrial—13%
  - ○ Sport—13%
  - ○ Other—12%
  - ○ Unknown—9%
- Age
  - ○ Mean—29 years
  - ○ Median—26 years
  - ○ Less than age 30—57%
- Work-related injuries
  - ○ 20% of all injuries
  - ○ 95% male
  - ○ Leading reported occupation—construction
  - ○ Leading cause—hammering metal or nails
- Initial vision
  - ○ 20/40 or better—17%
  - ○ 20/50–20/100—11%
  - ○ 20/120–1/200—15%
  - ○ HM—21%
  - ○ LP—23%
  - ○ NLP—13%
- Source of injury
  - ○ Blunt object—31%
  - ○ Sharp object—18%
  - ○ Motor vehicle crash—9%
  - ○ BB gun—6%
  - ○ Gun—5%
  - ○ Fall—4%
  - ○ Hammering metal on metal—5%
  - ○ Explosion—3%
  - ○ Fireworks—5%
  - ○ Nail—5%
  - ○ Unknown or other—9%
- Eye protection
  - ○ None—78%
  - ○ Regular specs—3%
  - ○ Safety specs—2%
  - ○ Unknown—15%
  - ○ Other—2%

Based on data from the United States Eye Injury Registry, 1998–2000.

tial visits presenting with NLP are due to assault. Drug and alcohol abuse, lower education, and lower income level have also been associated with increased numbers of violent ocular injuries.

The most common cause of serious ocular injuries is a blow caused by a blunt object. In the United States the primary culprits are fists, baseballs, rocks, and lumber. The large majority of victims were wearing no eye protection at the time of the incident.

CLASSIFICATION OF OCULAR TRAUMA

Historically, various systems have been used to classify ocular trauma. These have employed differing terminology and created confusion. For example, a "corneal penetrating injury" has been alternatively referred to as an injury penetrating only part of the cornea or as a full-thickness wound. Developed in 1994, the Birmingham Eye Trauma Terminology (BETT, Table 12–2) attempts to resolve this confusion by providing a definition for each type of injury and creating a standardized framework with which to classify the injury. BETT has been endorsed by a number of ophthalmological societies and organizations dealing with ocular trauma. It has become the standard system of clinical terminology used to describe ocular trauma.

> Open globe injuries have a full-thickness wound in the eye wall. Closed globe injuries do not.

The frame of reference is the entire eyeball, not

Table 12–2 Birmingham Eye Trauma Terminology (BETT)

Injury

- Closed globe: no full-thickness wound in eye wall (cornea or sclera)
  - Contusion: injury is due to direct energy of the object or from changes in the shape of the globe
  - Lamellar laceration: partial-thickness wound in eye wall. Wound is "into," but not "through"
- Open globe: full-thickness wound in eye wall
  - Laceration: caused by sharp object: injury by outside-in mechanism
    - Penetrating: entrance wound only
    - Perforating: entrance and exit wound caused by same object
    - Intraocular (retained) foreign body
  - Rupture: caused by blunt object: injury is caused by increase in IOP at vulnerable sites in eye—injury by outside-in mechanism

a specific part of the eyeball or the point where the object impacts the eye. All eye injuries are first classified into *closed globe* and *open globe* injuries. A full-thickness wound in the eyeball characterizes open globe injuries. Closed globe injuries have no full-thickness wound in the eye wall. The *eye wall* is defined as the cornea and sclera.

Closed globe injuries may be *contusions* or *lamellar lacerations*. In the case of a contusion, the damage results from the direct energy of the object or from changes in the shape of the globe (e.g., choroidal rupture or angle recession). A lamellar laceration is a wound "into," but not "through," the eye wall, as in the case of a corneal injury that penetrates only part of the stroma.

Open globe injuries cause full-thickness wounds in the eye wall. They are classified into *lacerations*, caused by sharp objects, and *ruptures*, caused by blunt objects. Lacerations are further divided into *penetrating*, resulting in a single (entry) laceration in the eye wall, *perforating*, resulting in two full-thickness (entry and exit) lacerations in the eye wall produced by the same object, and retained *intraocular foreign bodies*. (Technically intraocular foreign bodies are penetrating injuries but they are classified separately due to different clinical implications.)

In the case of a laceration the wound occurs at the impact site by an outside-in mechanism. In the case of a rupture the wound is caused not at the impact site itself but by an inside-out mechanism at another site. When the eye is struck, the intraocular pressure (IOP) rises and weaker points are preferentially damaged. An example of this would be a wound dehiscence of the cornea from prior cataract surgery even though the object has not directly struck this point. It is important to note that there may be some overlap in terminology and some injuries may be difficult to classify. Clinical judgment should be employed to choose the classification that best fits the case.

HISTORY

Obtaining a complete history plays an essential role in the examination, assessment, and management of the ocular trauma patient.

First and foremost, the clinician needs to obtain a detailed description of the traumatic event.

Ask patient to describe the traumatic event in detail.

Was the object striking the eye blunt, which would be expected to result in rupture, or sharp, leading to laceration? What was the speed of the offending object and from what distance did impact occur? The more force impacting upon the eye, the more damage would be expected.

In what type of environment did the trauma occur? If it occurred in a natural environment or one involving exposure to vegetable matter there is more likely to be microbial contamination. Was the patient wearing contact lenses, which would also place the patient at greater risk of infection? Was the patient wearing ocular protection, such as safety glasses? In the case of a motor vehicle accident, was the victim wearing a seat belt? Many accidents occur in the context of drug or alcohol use. The clinician should attempt to find out whether these substances were involved.

The nature of the object in contact with the eye needs to be determined. In the case of a chemical injury, was the substance acid or base? If there is any doubt as to the offending agent, the physician should obtain a sample.

Note the setting of the trauma, the nature of the object striking the eye, and the potential for infection.

The clinician needs to elicit the time of injury and whether the eye was getting better or worse. Certain burns such as those caused by basic chemical substances and ultraviolet radiation may produce relatively less pain initially and worsen with

Note patient symptoms and whether they are getting better or worse.

time. In these cases, the fact that the patient is not highly symptomatic upon presentation may not indicate the seriousness of the condition.

The physician should thoroughly investigate patient symptoms. Pain, photophobia, loss of vision, diplopia, flashes, and floaters may all be associated with trauma and contribute to the diagnostic picture. If there was loss of vision, did it occur immediately at the time of injury, or later? Hyphema may not cause reduction in vision initially, but will later in the event of a rebleed. Diplopia may be the result of an orbital floor fracture following extraocular muscle entrapment.

What actions did the patient take following the trauma? In the case of a burn, were the eyes irrigated immediately, and for how long? Did the patient use eyedrops? Drops such as vasoconstrictors may mask conjunctival hyperemia. Antibiotics or anti-inflam-

Ask patient what actions were taken in response to injury.

matory agents may influence the clinical presentation and healing process.

A complete ocular history should be obtained. The visual and health status of both eyes prior to the injury should be recorded. If the patient has a history of amblyopia in the traumatic eye, then reduction in vision in the injured eye may not entirely be due to the injury. Did the patient have a history of ocular surgery, which predisposes areas

Take ocular history. Note whether there was any prior problem with the traumatic eye.

of the eye to infection or wound dehiscence? Was there a prior injury to the eye, which might increase its vulnerability to further trauma?

The clinician needs to investigate the patient's medical history and determine how it impacts the clinical presentation. Blood disorders such as sickle cell anemia in addition to anticoagulant intake predispose the pa-

_____

Obtain a problem-oriented medical history.

_____

tient to increased risk of bleeding. Diabetes as well as inflammatory diseases such as rheumatoid arthritis can impair wound healing. Does the patient have any allergies, or a history of adverse reactions to any medication? The date of the last tetanus prophylaxis should be obtained. Open globe injuries may require the patient to receive an immune globulin or booster.

If ocular surgery is contemplated, the patient should be asked when his or her last meal was eaten. When the stomach is full, anesthesia creates the risk of pulmonary aspiration. If surgery is to be performed, the patient should be advised to eat no solid food for at least six hours prior to surgery. If surgery is uncertain, the patient should be instructed not to eat until the need for surgery has been determined.

Primary Actions—History Taking on Patient with Ocular Trauma

- Obtain detailed description of the traumatic event
- Determine the nature, force, and composition of the offending object
- Elicit actions taken by patient in response to trauma
  - Drops
  - Irrigation
  - Manipulation of eye
- Elicit patient symptoms
- Obtain complete ocular history including visual, health, and prior surgical status of both eyes prior to trauma
- Obtain complete medical history including medications, allergies, tetanus immunological status, and time of last meal

EXAMINATION OF THE TRAUMATIZED EYE

The examination of the patient with ocular trauma begins with the entire patient. It is important to remember that injuries to the eye may be associated with serious injuries to other parts of the body. The

_____

Check for serious systemic injury before examining eyes.

_____

patient's overall health status should be assessed and intervention should be taken, as appropriate. Only when a life-threatening emergency is ruled out should the examination proceed.

Visual Status

Best-corrected visual acuity (VA) should be obtained. In addition to the customary reasons, further importance is placed on this test in the event of ocular trauma due to possible litigation as a result of injury. Additionally, initial visual acuity is often a predictor of final visual acuity in cases of ocular trauma. Distance VA should be taken, but in cases in which this is impossible due to patient incapacitation, near VA should be taken. If vision is worse than 20/20 the patient should be refracted or pinhole vision should be taken.

Gross visual field testing by confrontation methods should be performed. Typically, more sophisticated testing by means of as automated or Goldmann perimetry is not needed at this point. Color vision may be assessed with tests such as pseudoisochromatic plates or the d-15.

Measure visual acuity and gross visual fields.

External Evaluation

The clinician should examine the lids and periocular area in bright light to look for signs of trauma. If an open globe is noted, the examiner should place a hard eye shield (not a pressure patch) over the patient's eye and orbital rim and immediately refer the patient for surgical repair.

The clinician should gently palpate the orbits and periocular area using sterile gloves, with eyes open in primary gaze. Care must be taken not to aggravate the injury. Look at the lids for signs of asymmetry. The clinician should try to determine whether there are any "step-offs," or irregularities and interruptions of orbital rim bones, suggesting fracture. Crepitus (or subcutaneous emphysema, suggesting a floor or medial wall fracture) and subcutaneous foreign bodies may be noted.

Other things to look for include contusions, ecchymosis, hemorrhage, loose bone fragments, edema, hyperemia, enophthalmos (recession of the eye in the orbit), exophthalmos (protrusion of the eye), ptosis, lacerations, and protruding foreign objects. Exophthalmometry should be performed if globe displacement is suspected. Palpation of the infraorbital area may reveal hypoesthesia, a sign of an orbital floor fracture. Supraorbital hypoesthesia suggests orbital roof fracture.

Examine periocular area. Note any irregularities of orbital rim, extrusion of ocular contents, crepitus, ecchymosis, or globe displacement.

The globe should be examined for the possibility of extruded ocular contents. Wounds should never be extended. Irrigation may be needed to rinse out an area to obtain a better view. If there is so much edema that the lids cannot be opened sufficiently to perform a proper exam, a speculum or lid retractor may be used to open the lids. However, care must be taken not to place too much pressure on the globe so as to increase the injury.

Documentation of the appearance of the injured eye should be made, either by way of a drawing or by photography. In addition to use for clinical purposes, this may be needed for instances of litigation.

Draw or photograph the injured eye.

Ocular Motilities

Extraocular muscle function should be evaluated in all fields of gaze. If there is restriction, forced duction testing should be performed. A positive forced duction test indicates muscle entrapment, hemorrhage, or orbital edema. A negative test is indicative of an oculomotor paresis or muscle evulsion.

Pupils

Pupils should be evaluated for response to light. Iris sphincter tears may result in dilated pupils. The swinging flashlight test should be performed to look for a relative afferent papillary defect (RAPD) indicative of optic nerve damage. If the pupil is not responsive due to the trauma, the optic nerve of the traumatic eye may still be evaluated for an RAPD by observing the other eye. If the noninjured eye dilates during the swinging flashlight test when the light is shone on the injured eye, then there is an RAPD in the injured eye. The reduction of the afferent signal in the injured eye results in a decreased efferent signal to the noninjured eye.

Evaluate EOMs and pupils, noting signs characteristic of ocular trauma.

Biomicroscopy

Slit-lamp examination should be performed to carefully examine the external and internal structures. Attention should be paid in looking for contusions, lamellar lacerations, full-thickness lacerations, ruptures, penetrating injuries, and foreign bodies. The anterior chamber should be examined for presence of hyphema and cells and flare. The iris should be examined for any sphincter tears, or iris dialysis (separation of iris from the root). If there is suspicion of an open

---
Perform biomicroscopy. Use Seidel test to check for full-thickness wound.

---

globe injury, a Seidel test needs to be performed to determine if there is a full-thickness corneal wound. The lens needs to be examined to note any displacement, phacodonesis (quivering of the lens with movement of the eye), cataract, or zonular rupture.

Gonioscopy

Gonioscopy is performed to examine angle structures, with special attention to angle recession (tear in the ciliary body) or cyclodialysis cleft (separation of the ciliary body from the scleral spur). Gonioscopy should not be performed in the case of hyphema as it may exacerbate bleeding.

> *Defer gonioscopy and scleral depression in cases of hyphema.*

Intraocular Pressure

Intraocular pressure should be measured. Depending upon the presentation, Goldmann tonometry may not be possible and pressure may need to be taken with a Tonopen or digitally. Low pressure is seen in cyclodialysis and choroidal detachment, and in some cases of anterior uveitis. High pressure may be an indication of aqueous outflow blockage.

Dilated Fundus Exam

A dilated fundus exam should always be performed to examine the vitreous and retina. Scleral depression should be deferred in the case of hyphema or with significant structural damage to the globe.

> *Perform DFE and order imaging tests as needed.*

Auxiliary Tests

Imaging studies such as plane X-rays, CT scan, and MRI may be employed as necessary.

Additional Considerations

Additional considerations often need to be made in the event of special populations such as children and the elderly. Children may not report wounds or underreport symptoms. Ocular damage may be a sign of child abuse. Should this be observed, it is incumbent upon the practitioner to notify the appropriate personnel.

Many injuries to the elderly result from falls. In these cases, the practitioner needs to be sensitive to the possibility of damage to other organs that may have life-threatening consequences. The possibility of dementia should also be noted. The clinician needs to work with family or other caregivers to coordinate patient management.

Primary Actions—Examination of Patient with Ocular Trauma

- Determine if there is an imminent life-threatening emergency
- Evaluate visual function
- Complete internal and external evaluation of eye
  - ○ Determine whether there is an open or closed globe injury
  - ○ Evaluate each ocular structure for damage characteristic of trauma
  - ○ Make a drawing or photodocumentation of injured area
- Provide attention to needs of special populations, such as children or elderly

OCULAR INJURIES—MANAGEMENT

Lids

Trauma to the lids is common. *Uncomplicated superficial lacerations* may be managed in the doctor's office. The area should be cleansed and irrigated, and a sterile dressing applied (Table 12–3). A topical antibiotic ointment should be applied three to four times a day. Oral antibiotic prophylaxis is not needed.

Manage superficial lid wounds with cleansing and antibiotic ointment.

Deeper or *complicated lacerations* need to be referred for surgical repair. In the case of an apparently contaminated wound or bite, antibiotic

Table 12–3 Management of Patient with Trauma to Lids

- Superficial or uncomplicated laceration
  - ○ Management in office with cleansing, antibiotic ointment, and dressing to wound
- Deeper or canalicular lacerations
  - ○ Referral for surgical repair
- Ecchymosis
  - ○ Cold compresses for first 24–48 hours, followed by warm compresses
- Ptosis
  - ○ Typically resolves spontaneously within 9 months; if not, surgical consult

prophylaxis is indicated. Tetanus prophylaxis should also be considered. Any patient with a tetanus-prone wound who has not had a booster shot within the last five years should be referred for prophylaxis. Rabies prophylaxis should also be considered in the case of animal bites.

Lacerations in the medial canthus may be associated with *canalicular lacerations*. The canalicular system should be examined by punctual dilation and irrigation. Leakage of fluid indicates canalicular damage. All canalicular lacerations need to be repaired.

> *Refer deeper lid wounds or canalicular wounds for surgical repair. Consider tetanus prophylaxis.*

Eyelid or canicular lacerations do not require immediate surgery and may be delayed for 24 to 48 hours so that appropriate arrangements may be made. Such surgery may take place in the surgeon's office, emergency room, or operating room depending upon the nature and extent of the injury.

In addition to lacerations, many lid injuries present as *ecchymosis*, often referred to as "a black eye." This results from subcutaneous hemorrhage and edema. The location of the lesion should be noted. Involvement of the lower lid and inferior orbital area may be suggestive of an orbital floor fracture. Ecchymosis should be treated with cold compresses for the first 24 to 48 hours followed by warm compresses several days afterward as needed.

> *Treat ecchymosis with cold compresses for the first two days, then warm compresses thereafter.*

Lid trauma may also result in *ptosis*. This is due to damage to the levator palpebrae muscle, such as from hematoma. This typically resolves in six to nine months. If the levator aponeurosis is stretched or torn, permanent ptosis may ensue, and surgery may be required to repair the damage.

Orbit

Orbital hemorrhage occurs from bleeding into the orbital space behind the globe and orbital septum. Blood may enter the extraocular muscle cone or the belly of an extraocular muscle. It may be present generally or locally within the orbit. Use of anticoagulants as well as systemic conditions such as hemophilia and platelet abnormalities may precipitate this in the event of minor trauma.

Signs for the examiner to look for include proptosis, subconjunctival hemorrhage, afferent papillary defect, motility restriction, increased IOP (due to orbital congestion), choroidal folds, central retinal artery pulsation, increased resistance of the globe to retropulsion, and globe displacement (Table 12–4). Symptoms include pain, nausea, vomiting, decreased vision, and diplopia.

Table 12–4   Management of Orbital Hemorrhage

- Observe for signs of proptosis, motility restriction, resistance to retropulsion, increased IOP, CRA pulsation
- Determine whether vision-threatening or non-vision-threatening
  - ○ If non-vision-threatening
    - ■ CT of orbits
    - ■ Cold compresses, head elevation, manage IOP if necessary
  - ○ If vision-threatening
    - ■ Treat CRAO if present
    - ■ Referral for orbital decompression

Orbital hemorrhage may compress and occlude the central retinal artery (CRA). This is an ocular emergency for which immediate action must be taken to increase the chance of preserving sight (see Chapter 17).

Traumatic orbital hemorrhage typically resolves spontaneously. Thus, *non-vision-threatening hemorrhages* may be monitored. A CT scan of the orbits with axial and coronal views should be performed. The patient should be treated with cold compresses and head elevation. IOP-lowering medications should be administered as necessary. Extraocular muscle restrictions usually resolve within a few weeks to nine months, depending on penetration of the hemorrhage.

Order CT scan in cases of suspected orbital hemorrhage.

Patients presenting with *vision-threatening hemorrhages* such as CRA occlusion, optic neuropathy, or intractably high IOP need to be referred for evaluation for decompression surgeries.

Orbital floor fracture, or blowout fracture, is commonly associated with blunt ocular trauma. It is likely to occur when an object larger than the size of the orbit strikes the eye. The inferior and medial walls of the orbit are most vulnerable to fracture in the event of trauma. Fracturing the orbit rather than the eyeball is thought to protect the globe from the increased pressure generated in response to the impact.

Ocular signs of an orbital floor fracture include motility restriction, particularly on superior gaze, enophthalmos, crepitus, and infraorbital hypoesthesia. The periorbital area should be palpated for crepitus and irregularity of the rim (Table 12–5). The patient may report diplopia. Restriction on eye movement occurs from orbital edema, hemorrhage, or muscle entrapment. Tissue herniation occurs into the maxillary and ethmoidal sinuses. Typically, entrapment of the inferior rectus results

Palpate orbital area for signs of fracture.

Table 12–5   Management of Orbital Fractures

- Orbital floor and medial wall
  - ○ Gently palpate orbital rim observing for irregularities
  - ○ Look for signs of enophthalmos, crepitus, inferior orbital hypoesthesia, restriction on eye movement
  - ○ Orbital CT scan if indicated
  - ○ Treat with broad-spectrum antibiotic for 10–14 days, ice packs, nasal decongestant
  - ○ Follow up in 7–10 days
  - ○ Surgical consult in case of complications or failure to resolve spontaneously
- Orbital roof fracture
  - ○ Observe for signs of exophthalmos, ptosis, ecchymosis in superior orbital area
  - ○ Note potentially serious sequelae due to proximity of cranium
  - ○ Refer for neurosurgical evaluation
- Lateral wall (tripod fracture)
  - ○ Observe for signs of enophthalmos, reduced sensation in lateral cheek, difficulties with mandibular movement
  - ○ Refer to facial surgeon

in restriction of upgaze, but restriction can occur in inferior and lateral gaze as well. Enophthalmos is due to expansion of orbital volume and may not be noted for a few days until edema resolves. Infraorbital hypoesthesia results from damage to the infraorbital nerve that travels in the floor of the orbit.

Signs and symptoms of an orbital blowout fracture often resolve spontaneously. There is some controversy as to whether a CT scan is routinely required. Orbital CT scan should certainly be performed if there is doubt about diagnosis, surgery is being considered, or there is suspicion of other orbital bone fractures.

> *Order orbital CT if diagnosis is uncertain or surgery is considered.*

A blowout fracture is not an ocular emergency. Management includes nasal decongestant for 10 to 14 days, ice packs for the first 24 to 48 hours, oral analgesics as needed, and broad-spectrum pro-

> *Manage uncomplicated blowout fractures with broad-spectrum antibiotics.*

phylactic oral antibiotics for 10 to 14 days, e.g., cephalexin (Keflex) 250–500 mg qid or erythromycin 250–500 mg qid. The patient should refrain from activities such as nose blowing, coughing, and sneezing, which raise sinus pressure and contribute to orbital emphysema. The patient should be seen for follow-up one to two weeks after the injury.

Indications for and timing of surgical repair are controversial and include

Refer complicated blowout fractures for surgical consult.

large fractures, persistent diplopia, cosmetically unacceptable enophthalmos, or "trap door" entrapment, a special kind of orbital floor fracture occurring when the inferior rectus herniates into the maxillary sinus and is pinched off by a bone fragment. Surgery should usually wait 10 to 14 days to allow edema to subside without risking fibrosis. Referral is to an ocuplastic surgeon.

The thin, *medial orbital wall* can be fractured in a similar fashion as the orbital floor. Orbital emphysema, caused by expulsion of air from the ethmoid sinus into the orbit, may result. Periorbital skin can inflate in the event of sneezing or nose blowing. Other signs include depressed nasal bridge and deviated nose, difficulty breathing if the nasal septum is damaged, and potential damage to the nasal lacrimal drainage system. As in the case of orbital floor fractures, the patient may present with enophthalmos and ocular motility restriction. Medial rectus entrapment is rare. Workup and management are similar to those of orbital floor fractures.

Manage medial wall fractures in similar fashion as blowout fractures.

Orbital roof fractures are uncommon due to bone thickness but much more serious than inferior or medial wall fractures due to proximity to the anterior cranial fossa. Patients will present with exophthalmos rather than enophthalmos, superior ecchymosis, and ptosis due to levator damage. Superior rectus entrapment can lead to restriction on depression.

Refer orbital roof fractures to a neuro-ophthalmologist or neurosurgeon.

Cerebral spinal fluid (CSF) can leak into the orbit and nasal cavity due to a direct communication of the orbit with the cranium. Additional potential complications include pneumocephalus, intracranial injury, CSF leak, meningitis, and abscess. The patient should be referred to a neurosurgeon.

Lateral wall fractures rarely occur, due to the thickness of the zygomatic bone. Fractures more commonly occur where the zygomatic arch meets its lateral and inferior orbital rim articulations at the frontozygomatic and zygomaticomaxillary sutures. This is known as a tripod fracture. Signs include limitation of mandibular movement, inability to open the mouth, enophthalmos, loss of prominent cheekbone, and hypoesthesia of the lateral cheek. The patient should be referred to a facial surgeon for evaluation and repair.

Ocular Burns

Thermal burns occurring to the lids may cause ocular complications from cicatricial scarring leading to entropion, ectropion, and trichiasis. First-degree burns involve only the epidermis. Sunburn is an example. Second-degree burns damage the epidermis and part of the dermis. Blisters form and the skin heals with minimal scarring in a few weeks. Third-degree burns involve the full thickness of the dermis, resulting in charring of the skin.

Manage mild lid thermal burns with cleansing, antiseptic, and antibiotic ointment.

First-degree lid burns may be managed in the optometric office. Signs and symptoms include pain to touch, erythema, and warmth. Management involves gentle removal of lid matter with gauze and saline, followed by an antiseptic application such as Povidone Iodine 5% ointment, avoiding contact with the eye. The patient should then be placed on a topical antibiotic ointment such as erythromycin two to four times a day and lubricants.

Thermal corneal burns have raised epithelial edges with an opaque gray appearance. They should be treated as an abrasion (see below).

Chemical burns constitute an ocular emergency for which immediate action is required. Permanent loss of vision may ensue. Alkali burns typically cause more damage than acid burns. The severity of the injury is related to the concentration of the substance and the extent of ocular penetration. Tissue penetration is greater with alkali than acid burns, which tend to cause more localized damage.

Signs include conjunctival hyperemia, chemosis, corneal clouding, epithelial erosion, stromal edema, and anterior chamber reaction. Alkali burns result in conjunctival blanching and limbal ischemia. Conjunctival vessel damage prevents corneal re-epithelialization since epithelial migration depends upon an intact conjunctival vascular response. Corneal opacification may result.

The eye should be irrigated immediately, for at least 30 minutes (see Table 12–6). If the patient phones for an appointment, he or she should be instructed to irrigate the eye copiously before coming into the doctor's office. If eyewash or sterile saline is not available, the patient may irrigate with tap water.

In the case of a chemical burn, irrigate eye immediately, prior to testing.

Table 12–6 Management of Chemical Burns

- Provide copious irrigation *immediately*, swabbing fornices for at least 30 minutes or until neutral pH
- Determine the nature of burn, alkali or acid. Alkali is more severe and associated with conjunctival blanching and corneal melt
- For mild burns—antibiotic ointment, frequent lubrication with nonpreserved artificial tears, and cycloplegia
- See patient the next day
- For severe burns, add topical steroid
- Severe burns should be referred to a corneal specialist after emergency treatment is employed

Check fornices for chemical particles. Determine pH of substance. Irrigate until neutral.

Upon presentation at the office, the eye should be irrigated before visual acuity is taken. The upper lid should be doubly everted, and all conjunctival fornices swept with a moist cotton tip applicator or glass rod to remove any remaining particles. Litmus paper should be applied to the conjunctiva to check pH. The irrigation process should continue until a neutral pH is achieved. The examiner should take the history after irrigation has begun. The offending agent should be inspected. Alkali burns may need to be irrigated for up to 48 hours after injury.

For mild corneal burns, the patient should be placed on an antibiotic ointment four times a day. Oral pain medication may be used if necessary. The patient should be instructed to lubricate copiously, with nonpreserved artificial tears every hour. Follow-up should occur the next day. Cycloplegia will reduce inflammation and pain from ciliary spasm. Steroid drops such as 1% prednisolone acetate every hour to every four hours may be used to treat more severe burns but should be tapered after the first 7 to 10 days in the event of a remaining epithelial defect due to risk of corneal melt.

Manage mild burns with topical antibiotic, cycloplegia, and anti-inflammatory medications.

Refer severe burns to corneal specialist.

Intraocular pressure may low (due to reduction in ciliary body output) or high (due to inflammatory debris blocking the trabecular meshwork or increased episcleral venous pressure). IOP-lowering drops such as beta-blockers or alpha-agonists should be employed.

In the case of more severe burns, referral to a corneal specialist is indicated after emergency treatment is employed.

Corneal abrasions (Figure 12–1) involve damage limited to the epithelium, the superficial layer of the cornea. The epithelium stains with fluorescein dye and may appear loose and bunched up. Staining presenting in a linear pattern may be caused by a scrape from a foreign object. Corneal abrasions should be differentiated from corneal ulcers, in which a stromal infiltration and excavation exist.

Patient symptoms include pain, foreign body sensation, and photophobia. There may be a history of trauma to the eye, as in the case of recurrent corneal erosion. The clinician should defer tonometry if it risks damaging the wound.

Patients with corneal abrasions should be treated with antibiotic prophylaxis (Table 12–7). Well-tolerated medications two to four times a day may be

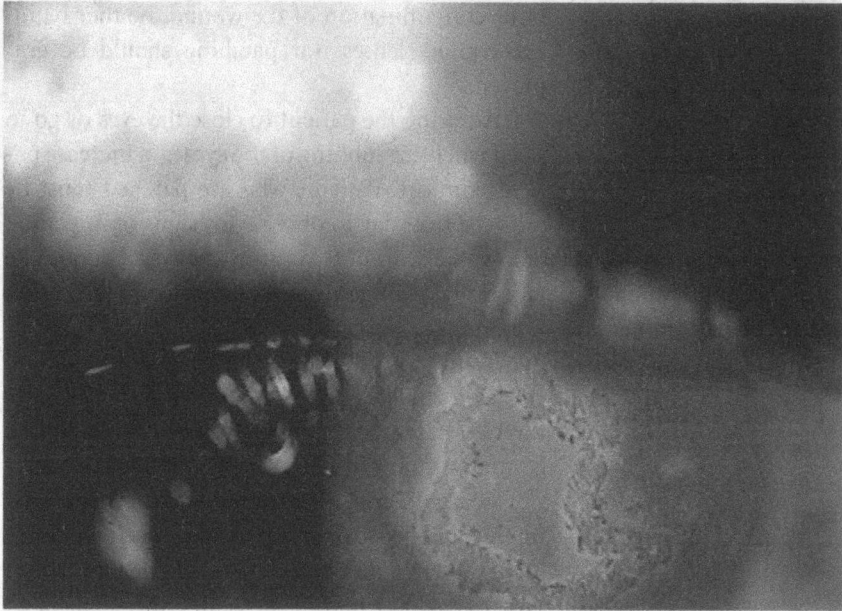

Figure 12–1. Corneal abrasion from a paper cut to the eye.

used. Nonsteroidal antibiotic drops can be used to reduce pain. Cycloplegia may be employed to reduce pain from ciliary spasm. For mild abrasions, it is often sufficient to give the patient a cycloplegic drop in the office rather than a prescription to use at home.

Manage mild abrasions with antibiotics, cycloplegia, and anti-inflammatory medications.

Pressure patching, more common in the past, is no longer used as a matter of course. In the case of a large wound or severe pain, a bandage contact lens may be employed. Disposable lenses work well. If there is a risk of infec-

Table 12–7   Management of Corneal Abrasion

- Observe for fluorescein staining
- Differentiate from corneal ulcer (no infiltrate present)
- Management
  - ○ Antibiotic ointment or drops
  - ○ Nonsteroidal anti-inflammatory and/or cycloplegic for pain
  - ○ Bandage contact lens or patching when indicated
  - ○ Advise patient to rest eyes
  - ○ Follow up within three days; next day if patched

Employ bandage contact lenses or patching for more severe abrasions when risk of infection is low.

tious contamination of the wound, neither bandage contact lenses nor patching should be employed.

Advising the patient to close the eyes or go to sleep will limit rubbing of the eyes and increase patient comfort. Patients who are patched must be seen the next day to observe for signs of infection. Patients who are not patched may be seen in two to three days. It should be remembered that diabetic patients take longer to re-epithelialize. Medication should be discontinued as healing takes place.

Evaluate for open globe injury by Seidel test and measurement of A/C depth.

Traumatic injuries to deeper layers of the cornea include *closed globe* injuries and *open globe* injuries. In the case of an open globe corneal injury, communication has been made between the anterior chamber and the external environment. Distinguishing between an open and closed globe injury is essential. A Seidel test should be performed. If there is aqueous leak, then an open globe injury is present. Other signs of an open globe injury include corneal hydrops, a rupture in Descemet's membrane leading to massive corneal edema. The depth of the anterior chamber should be evaluated. A shallow chamber will be seen in the case of an open globe injury due to an aqueous leak.

Superficial closed globe injuries may be managed with antibiotic drops, ointment, cycloplegia, and bandage contact lens or pressure patching (Table 12–8). Topical steroids should be avoided, as they will delay wound healing. The patient should be evaluated the next day. Deeper injuries may need to be sutured.

Table 12–8 Management of Corneal Stromal Injuries

- Determine whether open or closed globe injury
  - ○ Seidel test
  - ○ Evaluate cornea for edema and depth of anterior chamber
- Closed globe injury
  - ○ Manage with topical antibiotic, cycloplegia, pressure patch, or bandage contact lens
  - ○ Follow up next day
- Open globe injuries
  - ○ Small wound leaks
    - ■ Treat as closed globe injuries
  - ○ Large wound leaks
    - ■ Provide patient with eye shield and refer for surgical repair

Some small open globe injuries will self-seal. Injuries consisting of small corneal wounds with minimal aqueous leakage may be treated in the same fashion as lamellar lacerations. If the aqueous leak persists beyond 48 to 72 hours, the patient should be referred for surgical evaluation to close the wound.

> *Manage closed globe and self-sealing open globe injuries with antibiotics, cycloplegia, bandage CL, and pressure patching.*

In the case of a patient presenting with a significant open globe injury, an eye shield should be applied and the patient referred out immediately.

Anterior Chamber and Iris

Hyphema (Figure 12–2) is a layering or clot formed by erythrocytes in the anterior chamber. It is believed to occur in one-third of cases of serious trauma. It may occur from blunt or lacerating trauma. Vessels of the iris, ciliary body, or choroid rupture from internal pressure following impact or tear directly as a result of a lacerating injury.

Hyphema is usually self-limiting. A clot forms, reaches its maximum fullness within a week following the injury, and eventually dissolves as the hyphema resolves spontaneously. In other cases, secondary hemorrhage, or *re-*

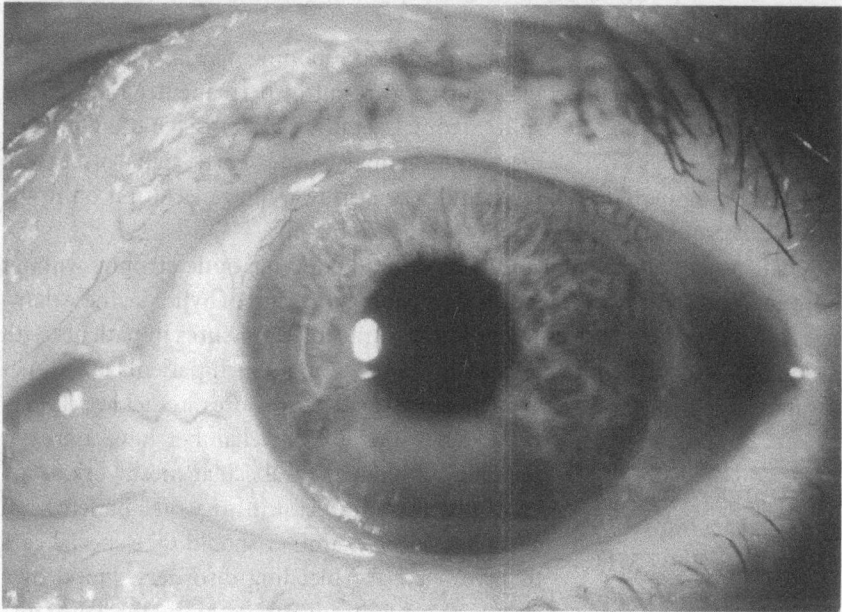

Figure 12–2. Hyphema from blunt trauma to the eye.

Note historical profile of patients at risk for hemorrhage.

bleeding, develops. This will result in an increase in the size of the hyphema and potentially lead to further complications. Visual prognosis is significantly worse in cases of rebleeds. A number of studies have found a higher rate of rebleeds in African-Americans. This may or may not be due to incidence of sickle cell hemoglobinopathy. Some studies have suggested it is attributable to increased iris melanin, which potentiates clot lysis. The risk of secondary hemorrhage also increases in patients with bleeding disorders and in those taking anticoagulant medication.

Grade the hyphema.

Grading systems have been devised to quantify hyphema. One is based on the volume of anterior chamber it comprises: Grade I < ⅓, Grade II ⅓–½, Grade III ½–less than total, Grade IV—total. Another is a measure in millimeters of the height of the blood layer. The blood can appear black in the case of a total hyphema. This is referred to as an "8 ball" hyphema.

Hyphema results in a number of complications. Increased intraocular pressure may occur due to occlusion of the trabecular meshwork or pupillary block. Total hyphema tends to be associated with high IOP. If IOP is normal or low in the event of a total hyphema, there should be concern about the possibility of an open globe. Anterior and posterior synechiae may develop due to inflammation and scarring.

Observe for corneal blood staining.

Corneal blood staining may last for years after the injury and result in permanently reduced vision. Stromal keratocyte necrosis and endothelial degeneration may ensue. Early signs of corneal blood staining include yellow granules or a straw-yellow discoloration in the posterior stroma, greater centrally than peripherally.

The potential exists for optic nerve head cupping, optic atrophy without cupping, and central retinal artery occlusion. As a result of hypoxia, these damages are more likely to occur with lower intraocular pressures in patients with sickle cell hemoglobinopathy than in those without. Such patients are also at an increased risk to develop higher intraocular pressures as sickle cell erythrocytes in the anterior chamber have a greater tendency to block the trabecular meshwork.

Observe for elevated IOP and possible consequences: ONH cupping and retinal vascular occlusions.

In performing a case history on a patient with a hyphema, the examiner should take special care to investigate for bleeding disorders, blood dyscrasias, thrombotic disorders, kidney and liver disease, anticoagulant therapy, and pregnancy status.

African-American patients should be tested for sickle cell disease by obtaining a sickle cell preparation and hemoglobin electrophoresis. Bleeding tests, including prothrombin time, partial thromboplastin time, platelet counts, and bleeding time, should also be performed on these patients.

Test African-American patients for sickle cell disease. Order bleeding tests.

A complete ocular health examination should be performed. The location and amount of hyphema should be measured. The cornea should be evaluated for blood-staining. The intraocular pressure needs to be measured at each visit, as it may vary depending on the course of the inflammatory response and the state of the hyphema. Gonioscopy and scleral depression may induce secondary hemorrhage and should be deferred for at least two weeks after the injury.

Perform complete ocular health exam. Defer gonioscopy.

Patient management (Table 12–9) is individualized and somewhat controversial. Goals are to promote clearing of blood and reduce the likelihood of rebleeds. Medical management includes, topically, atropine, 1%, one to three times a day and prednisolone acetate, 1%, four or more times a day as needed.

Manage with topical steroid and cycloplegia at minimum.

The antifibrinolytic agent aminocaproic acid may be used in an effort to delay clot lysis and reduce the incidence of rebleeds. Dosage is 50 mg/kg four times a day, up to 30 g/day for five days. Side effects include nausea, vomiting, and postural hypotension. The drug is contraindicated in some cardiovascular, renal, hepatic, and clotting diseases as well as in pregnant women. Man-

Table 12–9 Management of Hyphema

- Perform a complete medical history, with attention to blood dyscrasias, bleeding disorders, and current anticoagulant therapy
- Examination should stress evaluation for corneal blood staining, measurement of height of hyphema, and intraocular pressure
- Order laboratory tests as indicated
- Minimum treatment the first day includes
  ○ Cycloplegia
  ○ Topical steroid drops
  ○ Eye shield
  ○ Instruct patient to
    ■ Limit physical activity, elevate head while reclining
- Consider aminocaproic acid or prednisone po in severe cases
- Manage any elevation in IOP
- Determine whether hospitalization is necessary

When considering oral antifibrinolytic agent or steroid, comanage with ophthalmologist or patient's primary care physician.

Treat any elevation in IOP. Avoid prostaglandins and miotics.

agement should be coordinated with the patient's primary care physician. Following discontinuation of aminocaproic acid, clot lysis is likely to occur within the next three days. This may result in an increase in intraocular pressure. Prednisone 20 mg po bid may be used as an alternative to aminocaproic acid in high-risk patients.

The initial drug of choice for treating increased intraocular pressure associated with hyphema is a beta-blocker twice a day. If IOP is still elevated, alpha-agonists and topical carbonic anhydrase inhibitors should be used. Prostaglandins and miotics should be avoided. Acetazolamide (20 mg/kg/day up to a maximum of 250 mg qid) or methazolamide (10 mg/kg/day up to a maximum of 50 mg tid) may be used. Note that carbonic anhydrase inhibitors (which increase the risk of acidosis and sickling) and alpha-agonists (which affect iris vasculature) should be used with extreme caution in patients with sickle cell disease. If an oral carbonic anhydrase inhibitor is needed in a patient with sickle cell disease, methazolamide should be used, since there is less risk of acidosis than with acetazolamide. Patients with intractably high IOP require anterior chamber paracentesis or surgical removal of blood.

Hospitalize patients who are noncompliant or at high risk for rebleeds.

Upon disposition, give eye shield, advise to elevate head, and limit physical activity.

Patients with hyphema frequently need to be hospitalized. Those who are compliant adults, have low risk for secondary hemorrhage, have no history of blood diseases, with hyphema occupying less than one-half of the anterior chamber, with intraocular pressure less than 35 mm may treated on an outpatient basis.

Prior to leaving the office, the patient should be given a clear, rigid eye shield. Physical activity should be limited to minimal ambulation and the head should be elevated approximately 30 degrees while the patient is lying in bed. Any nonsteroidal anti-inflammatory medications, aspirin, or other anticoagulants should be discontinued. Oral acetaminophen may be used for pain. Patients who are not hospitalized should be seen the next day.

Anterior uveitis is common following ocular trauma. Symptoms include ocular pain and photophobia. The conjunctiva appears hyperemic and a ciliary flush is present. Increased vascular permeability and leakage of plasma proteins produce white blood cells and flare in the anterior chamber. In more severe cases a small amount of fibrin may appear in the anterior chamber. The intraocular pressure is usually low, likely due to decreased aqueous production by the ciliary body associated with inflammation, though increased outflow may play a part. A less common occurrence is increased intraocular pressure caused by

> *Manage traumatic uveitis with cycloplegic and/or topical steroid.*

restriction of aqueous outflow by inflammatory material. The pupil may be miotic.

Mild cases of traumatic uveitis may be treated with cycloplegia. They usually resolve within a few days. More severe cases may be treated with steroids, such as prednisolone acetate, 1%. The doctor should observe for anterior or posterior synechiae.

Iris

Traumatic iris structural damage includes *iris sphincter tears* (Figure 12–3) and *iridodialysis*. Sphincter tears result in the appearance of an angular-shaped irregularity at the pupillary margin. The pupil may be dilated and react poorly to light, either sectorally or across the entire circumference of the pupil.

> *Observe iris for sphincter tears and dialysis.*

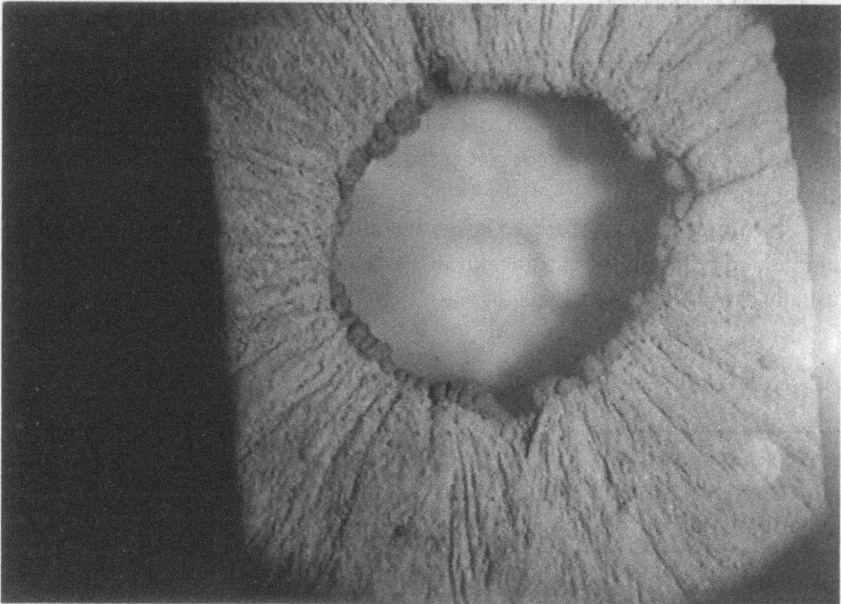

Figure 12–3. Iris sphincter tear after baseball injury to the eye.

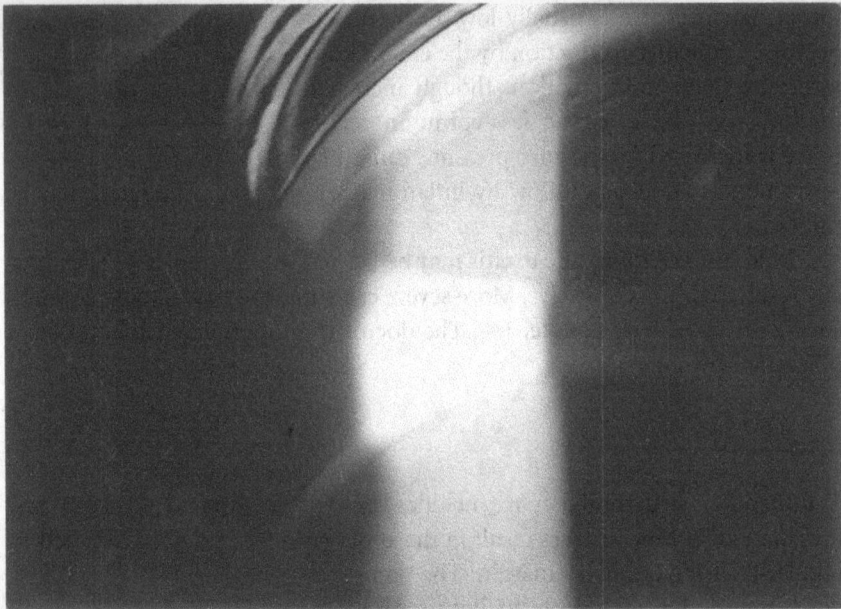

Figure 12–4. Angle recession in the same patient as Figure 12–3.

Consider clear-centered, opaque CL to manage diplopia.

Iridodialysis involves detachment of the iris from the root at the ciliary body. A large iridodialysis may create a displaced or multiple pupil leading to monocular diplopia. An opaque contact lens with a clear pupil may alleviate this, or the wound may be closed surgically. Patients with iris sphincter tears or iridodialysis should be evaluated closely for glaucoma because of frequently accompanying angle recession (Figure 12–4).

If trauma causes the iris to strike the anterior lens capsule, a permanent pigmented mark on the capsule, known as a *Vossius ring*, may be created. This usually causes no vision loss.

Angle Structures—Traumatic Glaucoma

Observe for signs of angle recession in patients with hyphema.

An *angle recession* is a rupture in the ciliary muscle between the circular fibers and the longitudinal fibers. It has been found in 70 to 100% of eyes with hyphema. Seven to nine percent of patients with angle recession develop glaucoma, in association with damage to the trabecular meshwork. Angle recession by itself will not elevate the intraocular pressure in the immediate aftermath of trauma. Glaucoma occurs later, sometimes by many years. It is therefore the task of the examining doctor at the time of trauma to evaluate the angle for the risk of glaucoma. Increased risk of developing glaucoma is associated with a larger area of recession.

Gonioscopy should be performed on all patients with potential for angle recession. The injured eye should be compared with the other eye to look for differences. Examination will reveal an

Perform careful gonioscopy.

enlarged, irregular ciliary body band. There may be torn iris processes. Pigmentary changes occur later.

Inflammatory glaucoma rather than angle recession glaucoma is more likely to occur in the immediate aftermath of ocular trauma. Inflammatory material or material from direct damage to ocular structures may block the angle. Outflow may also be impaired by inflammation to the trabecular meshwork itself. There may be anterior or posterior synechiae.

Management (Table 12–10) consists of prednisolone acetate, 1%, every hour to every four hours depending on the severity of the inflammation, cycloplegia, and a topical beta-blocker such as timolol, 0.5%, twice a day. If additional medications are

Manage any inflammatory IOP elevation with aqueous suppressant and topical steroid.

needed to lower IOP, Timolol .5%/Dorzolamide 2%, a beta-blocker–carbonic anhydrase inhibitor combination, may be used twice a day, or topical alpha-agonists such as Brimonidine .15% and Iopidine may be added twice a day. Oral carbonic anhydrase inhibitors and hyperos-

Table 12–10   Management of Angle Trauma

- Gonioscopy to evaluate for
  - ○ Angle recession
  - ○ Angle inflammation
  - ○ Synechiae
  - ○ Cyclodialysis cleft
- Treat any inflammatory glaucoma
  - ○ Prednisolone acetate, 1%
  - ○ Cycloplegia
  - ○ Topical beta-blocker
    - ■ Additional IOP-lowering agents as necessary
- Cyclodialysis cleft
  - ○ Marked initially by low IOP
  - ○ Cycloplegia
  - ○ Anti-inflammatory as needed
  - ○ Ophthalmological referral

motic agents may be used when there are no contraindications. Prostaglandins and miotics should not be used as they may exacerbate inflammation.

Angle Structures—Cyclodialysis Cleft

Place patient on cycloplegic drops. Refer to ophthalmologist to evaluate for surgical closure of cleft.

Gonioscopy may also reveal a cyclodialysis cleft following trauma. This is a tear between the longitudinal fibers of the ciliary muscle and the scleral spur. Aqueous fluid gains access to the suprachoroidal space resulting in very low IOP. The patient should be placed on a cycloplegic two to three times a day (Table 12–10). Ophthalmological referral should be made as closure may be needed by laser photocoagulation, cryotherapy, or suturing.

Lens

In eyes exposed to trauma, the lens should be examined for clarity, position, stability, and the integrity of the capsule (Table 12–11). Traumatic cataracts may result either from a penetrating object directly impacting the lens or via indirect damage from other intraocular structures.

Lens subluxation occurs in the event of partial or total dehiscence of the zonules from the lens capsule. Lens dislocation involves complete separation from the zonules. Signs and symptoms of a subluxated (Figure 12–5) lens include phaocodonesis and iridodonesis (wobbling of the lens and iris upon eye movement), visible zonules, glare, astigmatism, monocular diplopia, high myopia, and vitreous herniation into the anterior chamber. An ultrasound biomicroscope may be helpful in diagnosis.

Evaluate lens for subluxation, phacodonesis, and damage to capsule.

A dislocated lens may be positioned in the an-

Table 12–11 Management of Trauma to Lens

- Note formation of cataract
- Determine position of lens, i.e., subluxation or dislocation
- Determine whether capsule is intact
- Evaluate for phacolytic consequences
  - ○ Uveitis
  - ○ Glaucoma
- Evaluate for pupillary block and angle closure
- Manage intraocular pressure and inflammation
- Refer to cataract surgeon

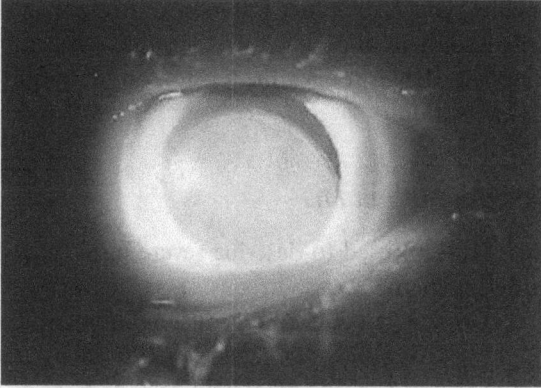

Figure 12–5. Subluxed lens from blunt trauma.

terior chamber or vitreous. Subluxated and dislocated lenses alone do not constitute an ocular
emergency if the capsule is intact and other structures, such as those of the angle, are not impinged
upon. The patient should be referred to a cataract

> *Refer dislocated lenses to
> cataract surgeon for
> repositioning.*

surgeon for repositioning. Lenses dislocated in the vitreous are sometimes left
in place in the case of an asymptomatic patient with no additional ocular complications.

If the lens capsule is broken, then the eye is subject to inflammation. Lib-
eration of lens particles may lead to phacolytic glaucoma. There is severe pain,
photophobia, injection, and edema, as extrusion of lenticular material and inflammatory cells accumulates in the aqueous, on the corneal endothelium, and
in the trabecular meshwork blocking outflow.

On an emergency basis, the immediate goal is to reduce intraocular pressure and inflammation prior to surgery. Medications to use include topical
beta-blockers, alpha-agonists, carbonic anhydrase
inhibitors, as well as systemic carbonic anhydrase
inhibitors and hyperosmotic agents if necessary.
Prostaglandins and miotics should be avoided.
Topical steroids and cycloplegic agents should be
used to reduce inflammation and increase patient
comfort. Referral should then be made to a cataract
surgeon.

> *Manage phacolytic events
> with aqueous
> suppressants, cycloplegia,
> and anti-inflammatory
> agents.*

Pupillary block may also result from a dislocated or subluxated lens. The lens or herniated vitreous may block the pupil, leading to angle closure.

> *Observe for signs of
> pupillary block.*

Again, the immediate goal is to reduce intraocular pressure and inflammation prior to definitive treatment of peripheral iridotomy or lens removal. Miotics should not be used, as they will relax the tension on the zonules, moving the lens further out of position.

Posttraumatic Endophthalmitis

Endophthalmitis is a term used to describe severe intraocular inflammation involving the anterior chamber and vitreous. It is usually caused by infection. It is an emergent condition, which may lead to rapid, permanent loss of vision. Trauma accounts for approximately 25% of cases of infectious endophthalmitis. Incidents following penetrating trauma range from 2.8% to 7.4% and are more prevalent in rural settings. Ocular foreign body injuries and those resulting from organic or contaminated material should alert the clinician to the potential of endophthalmitis.

> Be alert for signs of endophthalmitis with intraocular foreign body cases.

The most common causes of traumatic infectious endophthalmitis are *Staphylococcus aureus, Staphylococcus epidermidis, Streptococcus,* and *Bacillus cereus. Bacillus* accounts for 25% to 46% of traumatic endophthalmitis cases. Fungi are also sources. Multiple microorganism infections are not uncommon.

Symptoms include blurred vision, severe pain, conjunctival injection and edema, anterior chamber cell and flare, vitreous cells, hypopyon, and retinal periphlebitis. There may be vitreous infiltrates in the area of an intraocular foreign body. Fever may develop. A ring-shaped corneal infiltrate is characteristic of *Bacillus* endophthalmitis. Pain and inflammation often exceed what is expected from the traumatic event. Additionally, the vision may be worse than expected given the clarity of the media. Differential diagnosis includes severe inflammatory reaction to retained intraocular foreign body or proteins from ruptured lens (phacoanaphylactic endophthalmitis).

> Consider possibility of endophthalmitis when pain, inflammation, and reduction in vision exceed clinical expectations.

Workup includes culture and smears of aqueous and vitreous. B-scan as well as CT scan of the orbits to rule out the presence of intraocular foreign body may also be performed. The patient should be referred to a vitreoretinal specialist. Hospitalization is often required.

Medical treatment for traumatic endophthalmitis includes combinations of systemic, intraocular, and topical fortified antibiotics. Table 12–12 describes a common regimen. Steroids are not administered until an etiology of fungi

Table 12–12 Medical Treatment of Posttraumatic Endophthalmitis

- Topical (beginning on first postoperative day)
  - Vancomycin, 50 mg/mL q 1 hour
  - Ceftazidime, 50 mg/mL q 1 hour
  - Topical steroids and cycloplegics
- Periocular (subconjunctival)
  - Vancomycin, 25 mg
  - Ceftazidime, 100 mg
  - Dexamethasone, 12–24 mg
- Intravitreal
  - Vancomycin, 1 mg/0.1 mL
  - Ceftazidime, 2.25 mg/0.1 mL, or Amikacin, 0.4 mg/0.1 mL
  - Dexamethasone, 0.4mg/0.1 mL (optional)
- Systemic (usually reserved for more severe cases)
  - Vancomycin, 1 g iv q 12 hours
  - Ceftazidime, 1 g iv q 12 hours, or ciprofloxacin, 750 mg po q 12 hours for susceptible organisms

Source: American Society of Retinal Specialists.

can be ruled out. Surgical treatment includes vitrectomy, wound repair, and removal of any retained intraocular foreign body.

Treatment is usually not initiated at the optometrist's office.

Because diagnosis and treatment require surgical procedures, medical treatment is usually not initiated in the optometrist's office. Consultation should take place with the physician at the institution to which the patient is being referred to coordinate treatment. Antibiotic therapy is usually delayed pending specimen testing via anterior

Endophthalmitis cases require urgent consult with vitreo-retinal specialist.

chamber and vitreal tap or vitrectomy. However, because of the potential for rapid worsening of the eye, the referring doctor may be advised to commence treatment, particularly in rural settings where it may take the patient some time to arrive at the hospital.

Vitreous Hemorrhage

Red blood cells may appear in the vitreous as a result of torn retinal blood vessels. This may result in ghost cell glaucoma if there is a concurrent tear in the posterior capsule allowing the blood cells to obstruct aqueous outflow via the trabecular meshwork.

Perform B-scan to evaluate posterior segment when view of fundus is obstructed.

Table 12–13 Management of Vitreal, Retinal, and Choroidal Trauma

- Vitreal hemorrhage
  - ○ Determine whether retina is intact
    - ■ If not intact, refer for consult from retinal specialist
    - ■ If intact, may monitor. Bed rest, refrain from anticoagulants, follow up next day
- Retinal dialysis and detachment
  - ○ Determine whether macula is attached
    - ■ Macula attached—consult with retinal surgeon for surgery as soon as possible
    - ■ Macula unattached—arrange for consult with retinal specialist. Surgery may wait several days to one week. Advise bed rest.
- Choroidal detachment
  - ○ Initially treat with cycloplegia, e.g., atropine, 1%, three to four times a day and prednisolone acetate, 1%, four to six times a day.
  - ○ Refer for evaluation by retinal specialist

If the retina is not visible, B-scan ultrasonography should be performed to observe for signs of retinal detachment and any additional damage to the globe.

Advise patients with vitreous hemorrhage to have bed rest, elevate the head, and discontinue anticoagulants.

Patients with isolated vitreal hemorrhages due to trauma may be monitored initially (Table 12–13). Bed rest is advised, with elevation of the head to promote settling of the blood. The patient should refrain from using aspirin or other anticoagulants unless medically necessary. Follow-up should occur the next day.

Commotio Retinae

Also known as Berlin's edema (Figure 12–6), commotio retinae occurs minutes to hours after trauma. It presents as confluent white areas in the outer retina with ill-defined borders. It is thought to be due to a disorganization of photoreceptors, along with possibly intracellular retinal pigment epithelial edema. Any part of the retina can be involved. If the central retina is involved, it can cause reduced vision. No treatment is necessary, as the condition subsides over several weeks and vision typically returns to normal.

Patients with isolated commotio retinae may be monitored.

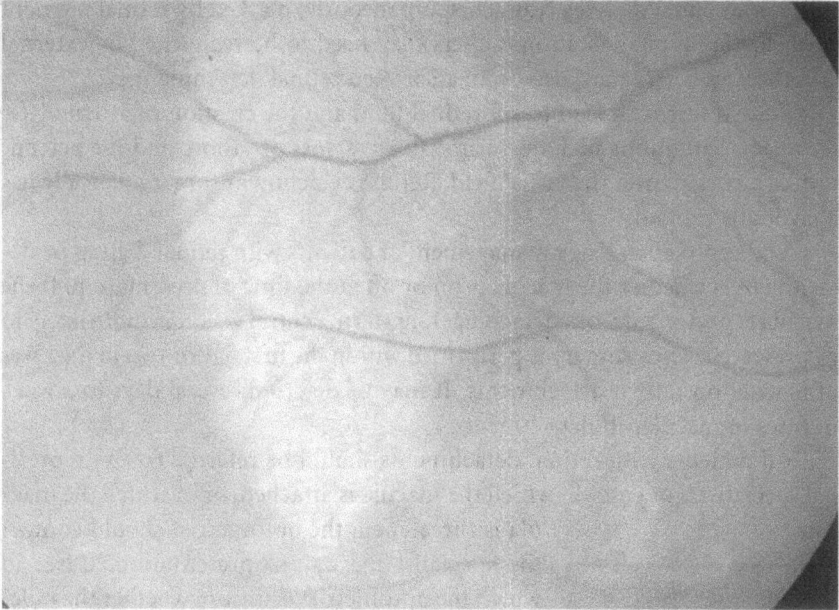

Figure 12–6. Commotio retinae (Berlin's edema) following retinal trauma.

Traumatic Retinal Defects

Retinal breaks occur when anterior-posterior compression of the eye results in lateral expansion of the globe in the equatorial region, resulting in vitreoretinal traction.

There may be avulsion of the vitreous base, retinal dialysis, tears, holes, and detachments. The vitreous should be carefully examined for pigmented cells, which are signs of breaks in the retina.

Retinal dialysis is a disinsertion of the peripheral retina from its attachment at the ora serrata. It is the most common retinal break associated with blunt trauma. The retina and pars plana tissue appear as a raised ridge in the anterior and posterior portions of the vitreous base. The most common retinal areas where this occurs are inferotemporal and superonasal. This is because the globe is least protected by the orbit in these areas. It is thus more vulnerable to an object striking from this direction. Patients with traumatic retinal breaks should be referred to a vitreoretinal specialist for evaluation. (See Chapter 18.)

Refer patients with traumatic retinal breaks to vitreoretinal specialist.

Some retinal dialyses reattach spontaneously, marked by retinal pigment epithelial hyperpigmentation. Others may need to be reattached by external cryotherapy. There may also be an associated retinal detachment.

Retinal tears can lead to subretinal fluid and the creation of a *retinal detachment*. Symptoms include flashes, floaters, loss of vision, and the perception of a curtain over the visual field. Retinal detachment surgery typically has a favorable prognosis.

The key to emergency management of patients with retinal dialysis or detachment is whether the macula is on or off at the time of presentation. If the macula is prevented from detaching, long-term central vision is more likely to be preserved. Thus surgery is performed within the first day or two in the cases of macula-on retinal detachments. It may be deferred several days to a week in cases of macula-off detachments.

All patients with retinal detachments should be referred to a vitreoretinal specialist. For cases in which the macula is attached, or in which the macula is threatened, the optometrist should contact the specialist the day of presentation. Cases in which the optometrist is unsure whether the macula is on should be treated as macula-on cases. If surgery is deferred, these patients should be advised to have bed rest until surgery.

Refer macula-on detachments immediately. Macula-off detachments are less urgent.

Vitreal traction may also result in a *traumatic macular hole,* but not usually upon initial presentation. Macular cysts appear initially, then rupture of the cysts creates macular holes, sometimes years later. Patients with macular cysts may be monitored. Patients with macular holes should be referred to a retinal specialist.

Traumatic Choroidal Defects

Choroidal detachments often result from blunt trauma or penetrating injury to the eye. They appear as bullous, smooth, lobular elevations of the retina and choroid and may extend for 360 degrees. Pressure surrounding choroidal vessels is rapidly decreased following the blow to the eye. Dilation of choroidal vessels ensues.

Choroidal detachments may be serous or hemorrhagic. Rupture within posterior ciliary arteries creates a hemorrhagic detachment, resulting in the accumulation of blood in the suprachoroidal space. Serous detachments transilluminate and are associated with very low intraocular pressure. The patient may be asymptomatic. Hemorrhagic detachments do not transilluminate and are associated with high intraocular pressure. The patient more often presents with a painful, red eye and reduced vision. Both cases present with a shallow anterior chamber and cell and flare.

> *Treat choroidal detachments with cycloplegia and topical steroids. Obtain vitreoretinal consult.*

Most choroidal detachments do not require immediate surgery. In the emergency setting, patients should be started on cycloplegic drops such as atropine, 1%, three times a day and steroidal anti-inflammatory drops such as prednisolone acetate, 1%, four to six times a day (Table 12–13). A retinal consult should be obtained, as surgical drainage may be required in a number of cases. Such cases include those presenting with flat anterior chambers, intraocular pressure greater than 30 mm, severe pain, and "kissing choroidals" (two choroidal lobules in apposition).

Choroidal rupture (Figure 12–7) results from indirect trauma following compression and horizontal lengthening of the globe. The globe recovers its original shape via oscillations. This causes a stretching of the ocular tissue resulting in injury to the retina, choroid, vitreous, optic nerve, and sclera. The relative inelasticity of Bruch's membrane makes this structure particularly vulnerable to rupture. It is accompanied by a disruption of the overlying RPE and underlying choriocapillaris.

The appearance of the choroidal rupture consists of a crescent-shaped scar, concentric with the optic disc, usually appearing in the macula area. There

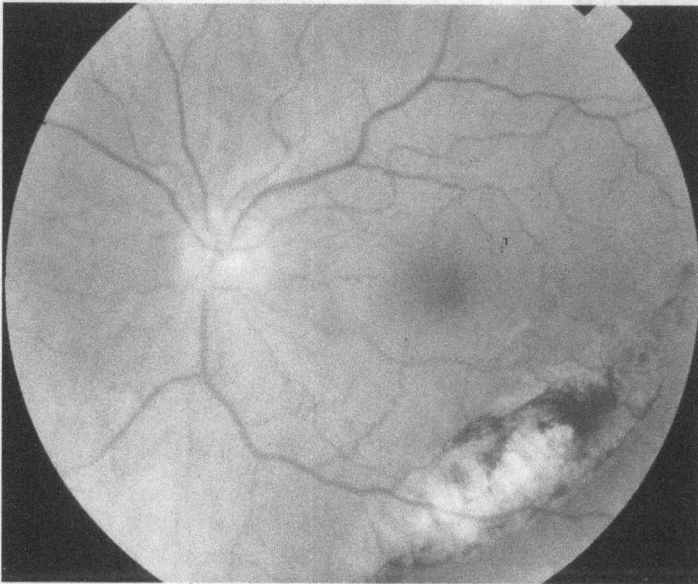

Figure 12–7. Choroidal rupture associated with blunt trauma.

Monitor patients with choroidal rupture for subretinal neovascularization.

is an initial hemorrhage, and the eventual formation of a yellow-white streak at the level of Bruch's membrane. Visual acuity is often reduced to worse than 20/200. The patient needs to be monitored for subretinal neovascularization, which may occur years following the injury.

Traumatic Optic Neuropathy

An object impacting the eye may penetrate the orbit and directly damage the optic nerve, or indirect forces may damage the nerve. In the latter case, blunt trauma causes sudden movement of the globe resulting in shearing or compression of the nerve by surrounding tissue, bone, or inflammation.

In the case of anterior traumatic optic neuropathy, the damage is to the intraocular or anterior orbital portions of the nerve. There may be a tearing at the lamina cribrosa and an associated hemorrhage or "optic nerve avulsion" (Figure 12–8). The disc will appear hyperemic, swollen, and surrounded by flame-shaped hemorrhages.

In posterior traumatic optic neuropathy, the damage is to the posterior orbital, intracanalicular, or intracranial portions of the nerve. The optic disc appears normal. Pallor does not occur until weeks later.

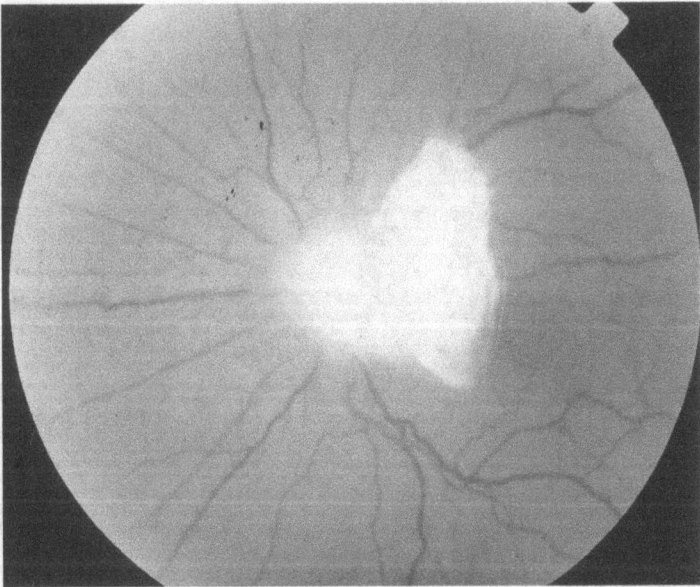

Figure 12–8.   Optic nerve avulsion.

In any case of traumatic optic neuropathy, the examiner should look for a relative afferent pupil defect, reduced color vision, desaturation to red hue, and reduced vision. Visual field testing should be performed. Management includes hospitalization, CT scan, systemic antibiotics, intravenous steroids, and optic nerve surgical intervention. A referral to a neuro-ophthalmologist is indicated.

> *Afferent pupillary defect, color vision defects, and disc hemorrhages are signs of traumatic optic neuropathy. Refer to neuro-ophthalmologist.*

Primary Actions—Assessment and Management of Patient with Ocular Trauma

- Determine the degree of urgency of the problem
- Determine whether treatment should be initiated by the optometrist or by a consulting doctor
- Provide or refer for treatment as appropriate

Chapter 13

Diplopia

"Doctor, I noticed all of a sudden I'm seeing double."

SCOPE OF THE PROBLEM

Diplopia, or double vision, can be one of the most disturbing of visual complaints. While many patients have experienced episodes of blurry vision, the alarm generated by the perception of two simultaneous images is uniquely disconcerting. Diplopia presents as a state of visual *confusion*, in which the patient sees two images and is unable to determine which represents the true location of the object. If it occurs during potentially hazardous activities such as driving, diplopia may have severe or life-threatening consequences. Moreover, diplopia is often a sign of serious systemic illness, such as neurological or vascular disease.

Diplopia has a wide variety of causes. It may be monocular or binocular (Tables 13–1 and 13–2). Monocular diplopia usually results from media aberrations or opacities. It may occur in both eyes simultaneously. Binocular diplopia usually results from misalignment of the visual axes. It may also occur in anisometropia, as a result of different images to each eye.

HISTORY

In taking a history, there are a number of important questions that need to be asked. The first is what the patient means by "double vision." Not infrequently, the patient will report "seeing double," when in fact he or she is describing a type of blur. The patient should be asked whether two separate objects are seen or one unclear object is seen. Sometimes the distinction between blur and diplopia is difficult to make. The patient may

Clarify what the patient means by "double vision."

Table 13-1   Major Causes of Monocular Diplopia

- Media abnormalities
  - ○ Corneal
    - ■ Keratoconus
    - ■ Corneal edema
    - ■ High astigmatism
    - ■ Ocular surface disease
    - ■ Deformation by swollen lid
  - ○ Iris
    - ■ Peripheral iridectomy
    - ■ Polycoria
  - ○ Lens
    - ■ Cataract
    - ■ Subluxated lens
- Macular disease associated with traction
- Cerebral abnormalities
  - ○ Polyopia
  - ○ Palinopsia
- Functional (nonorganic) causes

describe seeing two of the same objects overlapping, instead of two separate objects. Sometimes this is described as a ghost image or halo. This can occur in monocular diplopia as a result of media opacity.

The clinician should ask the patient whether the double vision disappears when one eye is covered. If it does, then the diplopia is binocular. If not, the diplopia is monocular. If it is monocular, the doctor must think in terms of ocular media etiologies. There are other causes such as macular or cerebral abnormalities but these are much less common.

Ask whether the double vision disappears when one eye is covered.

Another differential between binocular diplopia and monocular diplopia involves the clarity of the images. In the case of binocular diplopia, the images are typically equally clear. In the case of monocular diplopia one of the images is often faded or indistinct.

If the diplopia is binocular, additional questions need to be asked. Are the two images side by side, above and below each other, or obliquely oriented? Is the diplopia worse in right or left gaze? Is it worse at distance or near? These questions will help in determining which extraocular muscle(s) are involved in causing it. For example, horizontal diplopia, which is greater at distance, should alert

Ask whether the objects are located one on top of the other or side by side.

Table 13–2 Major Causes of Binocular Diplopia

Incomitant

- Isolated cranial nerve palsies
  - ○ Third
  - ○ Fourth
  - ○ Sixth
- Brainstem disorders
  - ○ Duane's syndrome
  - ○ Millard-Gubler syndrome
  - ○ Foville's syndrome
- Superior orbital fissure/cavernous sinus disorders
  - ○ Tolosa-Hunt syndrome
- Cerebral pathway disorders of ocular coordination
  - ○ Skew deviation
  - ○ Internuclear ophthalmoplegia
- Posterior fossa disorders
  - ○ Cerebellopontine angle tumors
- Chronic progressive external ophthalmoplegia
- Botulism
- Myasthenia gravis
- Thyroid ophthalmopathy (Graves' disease)
- Muscle entrapment due to orbital trauma
- Brown's superior oblique tendon sheath syndrome
- Toxic drug reactions

Comitant

- Decompensated phoria
- Strabismus
- Convergence insufficiency
- Accommodative or converge spasm
- Anisometropia/aniseikonia

the doctor to the possibility of sixth nerve palsy. Vertical diplopia may be caused by fourth nerve palsy or a decompensated vertical phoria. Diplopia consisting of obliquely oriented images may be the result of multiple cranial nerve involvement.

> *Ask whether the images are farther apart (1) at distance or near and (2) in right or left gaze.*

It should be ascertained whether the diplopia is constant or intermittent. If it is intermittent, when is it most likely to occur? Conditions such as myasthenia gravis create diplopia that is intermittent and variable. Different muscles may be involved on different occasions. It is worse

Ask about the frequency and conditions in which the diplopia occurs.

with muscle fatigue, and is thus likely to occur with activity and later in the day. Double vision occurring during the course of prolonged near-work is suggestive of convergence insufficiency or accommodative spasm.

Ask if there is a history of ocular or head trauma. Head trauma is the most common cause of fourth nerve palsies. Orbital trauma may result in horizontal or vertical diplopia.

The clinician also needs to determine whether the symptoms occurred suddenly or gradually. Diplopia of sudden onset points in the direction of vascular disease, such as diabetes or hypertension, which lead to cranial nerve infarction. Symptoms of gradual onset are suggestive of compressive etiologies such as thyroid ophthalmopathy.

Any systemic symptoms associated with the diplopia need to be noted. Symptoms such as proximal limb weakness, fatigue, or difficulty swallowing or breathing that occur late in the day are suggestive of myasthenia gravis. Ocular pain may be indicative of an extraocular muscle paresis caused by ischemia, aneurysm, orbital inflammation, or tumor. Neurological symptoms such as paresthesias may be associated with multiple sclerosis. Episodes of transient vision loss and motor difficulties may be associated with cerebral vascular disease.

Ask about rapidity of onset of diplopia and accompanying symptoms.

A full medical history needs to be obtained. Hypertension, diabetes, atherosclerosis, and giant cell arteritis are all associated with cranial nerve palsies due to vasculopathic etiologies. Thyroid disease is a common compressive cause of extraocular muscle restrictions resulting in binocular diplopia.

Obtain full medical history with attention to diseases that can cause extraocular muscle dysfunction.

The medical history should include the question of whether there are any current illnesses present. Diplopia resulting from a decompensated phoria may occur in the case of an acute illness or head trauma. Patient medications should be listed for possible associations with diplopia.

Primary Actions—Case History on Patient with Diplopia

- Distinguish between blur and diplopia
- Investigate whether diplopia is monocular or binocular
  - Ask whether diplopia disappears when one eye is covered
  - If binocular, ask whether diplopia is worse at distance or near, on right or left gaze, and about the position of the images in space

- Investigate the pattern of symptoms:
  - ○ Constant or intermittent
  - ○ Circumstances under which symptoms occur
  - ○ Gradual or sudden onset
- Determine whether there are any concomitant ocular or systemic symptoms
- Obtain full medical history with attention to conditions known to cause diplopia

EXAMINATION

One of the aims of testing is to determine the origin of the diplopia. The first determination the examiner must make is whether the diplopia is monocular or binocular. As noted above, if the second image does not disappear when one eye is covered, the diplopia is characterized as monocular.

> **Determine whether the diplopia is monocular or binocular.**

Monocular Diplopia

Once monocular diplopia is established, a pinhole test should be performed on the symptomatic eye. A multiple pinhole occluder is often easier for the patient to employ than a single pinhole. If the diplopia disappears with the introduction of the pinhole, then the diplopia is due to an ocular media abnormality. Such abnormalities, which produce multiple retinal images, create multiple images in space. In this case, refraction should be performed to see whether fully correcting the refractive error eliminates the symptoms.

> **Perform pinhole test on all patients with monocular diplopia.**

Should refraction fail to resolve the diplopia, the clinician then needs to examine the ocular media for diplopia-inducing abnormalities. Corneal etiologies include keratoconus, edema, high astigmatism, ocular surface disease, and deformation by swollen eyelids. Iris abnormalities include peripheral iridectomy and polycoria. Lenticular anomalies include cataract and dislocated lens.

> **Look for media abnormalities in patients with monocular diplopia.**

If the diplopia does not resolve with pinhole, then macular or neurological disease must be considered. If macular disease is suspected, an Amsler grid should be performed. Any perception of metamorphopsia by the patient should be noted.

Monocular diplopia of cerebral origin includes cerebral polyopia and palinopsia. A patient with polyopia perceives multiple copies of the same image. In the case of palinopsia, differing images are superimposed. The patient is unable to erase a visual image. The image persists, creating a superimposition with a different image seen later in time. Both polyopia and palinopsia are associated with occipitoparietal disease and occur in the presence of other symptoms. The patient should be referred for neurological workup.

Binocular Diplopia

Binocular diplopia occurs (assuming normal retinal correspondence) when the eyes point to a different direction in space. The extraocular muscles do not direct the foveae toward the same position. The condition may occur as a result of mechanical limitation to the muscle itself or because of damage along the neurological pathway that innervates the muscle. Testing should establish which muscle(s) are involved.

Extraocular Muscles

The following is a brief review of the actions of the six extraocular muscles and the cranial nerve (CN) that innervates them (Table 13–3): Horizontal movements are controlled by the lateral rectus (CN VI) for abduction, and the medial rectus (CN III) for adduction. Vertical movements are controlled by four muscles: the superior rectus (CN III) for elevation primarily in abduction, the inferior rectus (CN III) for depression primarily in abduction, the inferior oblique (CN III) for elevation primarily in adduction, and the superior oblique (CN IV) for depression primarily in adduction. Intorsion is controlled by the superior rectus primarily in adduction and superior oblique primarily in abduction. Extortion is controlled by the inferior rectus primarily in adduction and the inferior oblique primarily in abduction.

> *Ocular motilities are controlled by cranial nerves III, IV, and VI.*

One key in determining which muscles are involved in creating the ocular misalignment is the patient's head posture. The examiner should observe the patient for any evidence of compensatory head turn, head tilt, or vertical chin movement (Table 13–4). Compensatory head movements usually act to reduce the amount of diplopia. However, in some instances the head may be directed in the opposite direction, so as to increase the separation of the images in order that one may be more easily suppressed.

> *Observe patient for signs of head turn, head tilt, or chin positioning.*

Head turns compensate for horizontal misalignment. Vertical head move-

Table 13-3 Actions of Extraocular Muscles

Muscle	Cranial Nerve	Primary Action	Secondary Action	Tertiary Action
Lateral rectus	VI	Abduction		
Medial rectus	III	Adduction		
Superior rectus	III	Elevation (lateral gaze)	Intorsion (medial gaze)	Adduction
Inferior rectus	III	Depression (lateral gaze)	Extorsion (medial gaze)	Adduction
Superior oblique	IV	Intorsion (lateral gaze)	Depression (medial gaze)	Abduction
Inferior Oblique	III	Extorsion (lateral gaze)	Elevation (medial gaze)	Abduction

ment (chin position) compensates for vertical misalignment. Head tilt compensates for torsional misalignment.

Comitant and Incomitant Deviations

The examiner needs to distinguish between a *comitant* deviation, in which the angle of deviation is the same in all gazes, and an *incomitant* deviation, in which the angle varies with the direction of gaze. Comitant deviations tend to occur in congenital conditions. Incomitant deviations are more likely to occur in acquired disease.

> *In cases of comitant deviations, suspect congenital disease. With incomitant deviations, suspect acquired disease.*

There is a large variety of conditions that cause comitant and incomitant deviations. The most common comitant causes of diplopia are strabismus, decompensated vertical phoria, and convergence insufficiency. The most common incomitant causes are cranial nerve palsies (third, fourth, and sixth) (Fig-

Table 13-4 Compensatory Head Movements, Left Eye

Paretic muscle (OS)	Head turn	Head tilt	Chin position
Lateral rectus	Left		
Medial rectus	Right		
Superior rectus	Right	Right	Up
Inferior rectus	Right	Left	Down
Superior oblique	Left	Right	Down
Inferior oblique	Left	Left	Up

Adapted from Walsh, *Neuro-Ophthalmology: Clinical Signs and Symptoms*, 1997.

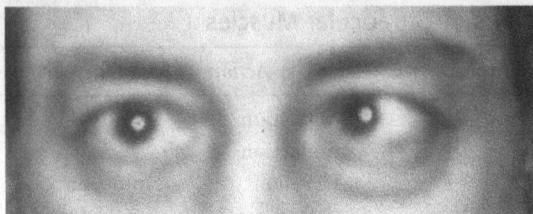

Figure 13–1. Sixth cranial nerve palsy.

ure 13–1), myasthenia gravis, trauma, and restrictive orbitopathies such as Graves' disease.

Binocular Testing

The following tests should be performed as needed on any patient with binocular diplopia: versions, ductions, distance, and near cover test, Maddox rod or red lens, and Park's three-step test. The amount of deviation should be measured in free space and neutralized with prism. Risley prisms in the phoropter are not recommended as they are designed for measurement in primary gaze.

Versions and ductions should be performed to evaluate the position of the globe in all nine cardinal positions of gaze. Any restriction or lack of comitancy should be noted.

Perform versions and ductions, noting comitancy.

The amount of misalignment found during the cover test will vary according to which eye is covered. When the test is performed on a patient with a comitant deviation, the angle of deviation will be the same regardless of whether the nondeviating eye is fixating (known as the primary deviation) or the deviating eye is fixating (known as the secondary deviation). In the case of incomitant deviations, the deviation will be greater when the deviating—in this case paretic—eye is fixating. This is because greater innervation is required for the paretic eye to fixate. The result is an increased signal to the nonparetic eye, thereby increasing the angle of deviation between the two eyes.

Sometimes the amount of incomitancy decreases over time. Modifications are made in the actions of both ipsilateral and contralateral muscles, resulting in the strabismus becoming more symmetrical. Known as a "spread of comitance," this is seen as an adaptive mechanism and is thought to be under cerebral control.

Perform cover test, noting primary and secondary deviations.

An isolated horizontal muscle palsy is relatively easy to diagnose. The patient reports two images side by side and limitation is noted on lateral gaze. The most common culprit is a sixth nerve palsy to the lateral rectus muscle. The patient will show eso posture at distance. If limitation is on medial gaze, the medial rectus is involved. In cases of ocular nerve palsies this is typically not observed in isolation. Since CN III innervates several extraocular muscles, movement will be restricted in other fields of gaze. Therefore, if the eye cannot adduct, but has full range of movement in all other fields of gaze, the problem is more likely due a mechanical restriction.

> *An isolated, unilateral abduction deficit is most commonly a sixth nerve palsy.*

If a vertical deviation is noted, testing becomes more complex. Four muscles, the superior and inferior recti and the superior and inferior oblique, are involved in vertical eye movements. A Park's three-step test should be performed to identify the affected muscle. The test involves noting any change in deviation of visual axes in differing positions of gaze.

Park's three-step test can be performed in a number of ways: objectively, by observing the corneal reflex from a transilluminator, as the eyes track an object in different fields of gaze, or subjectively, by breaking fusion and asking the patient to report on the positions of the two images. This is most commonly performed with a red lens or a red Maddox rod placed over one eye (conventionally the right). Nothing is placed over the other eye. A white muscle

> *Perform Park's three-step test on all patients with vertical deviations.*

light is directed toward the patient. When the red lens is used, the patient will see one red light and one white light. When the Maddox rod is used, the patient will see a red streak from one eye (perpendicular to the direction of the cylinders of the Maddox rod) and a white spot of light from the other eye.

The patient first focuses in primary gaze (Table 13–5). In the case of the red lens test, if a vertical deviation is present, the patient will see a white light and red light, one on top of the other. If a Maddox rod is used, the red line and white spot will be above or below one another. The direction of the image in space will be opposite to the position of the eye. For example, if

> **Step 1:** *Ask patient position of images in primary gaze.*

the red light is seen below the white light, the right eye is *above* the left eye.

In this example, there are four possibilities. The right superior oblique (RSO) or right inferior rectus (RIR) is not depressing the right eye. Or the left inferior oblique (LIO) or left superior rectus (LSR) is not elevating the left eye.

The next step will further serve to narrow down the choice of the affected muscle. The patient is asked whether the images are further separated in right or left gaze. Of the four muscles noted,

> **Step 2:** *Ask whether separation of images is greater in left or right gaze.*

Table 13–5 Park's Three-Step Test with Red Lens Covering Right Eye

Step	Gaze	Deviation	Possible muscles affected
1	Primary	White image higher	RSO RIR, LIO, LSR
2	Horizontal	Greater in left gaze	RSO LSR
3	Head tilt	Greater toward right side	RSO

those responsible for vertical movement in right gaze are the RIR and LIO. In left gaze they are the LSR and RSO. If the diplopia increases on left gaze, then either the RSO is not depressing the right eye, or the LSR is not elevating the left eye.

To determine which of these two muscles is involved, the Bielschowski head tilt test is performed. The separation of images is compared upon right and left head tilt. When the head is tilted right, the

Step 3: Compare separation of images on right and left head tilt.

RSO intorts the right eye. When the head is tilted left, the LSR intorts the left eye. If the deviation is greater on right head tilt, then the involved muscle is the RSO.

As a compensatory mechanism, patients with acute fourth nerve palsies often present with a head tilt toward the shoulder opposite the eye with the palsy. Thus, a patient with a right superior oblique palsy will tilt the head toward the left shoulder.

To distinguish between congenital and acquired fourth nerve palsy, vertical fusional ranges should be performed. The ranges will be larger in the case of congenital fourth nerve palsy, as a result of the patient having developed larger ranges to compensate for misalignment. Normal fusional ranges are 2–3 prism diopters. Patients with congenital fourth nerve palsies may have ranges as high as 10–15 prism diopters.

Another important method in determining whether the deviation is recent or long-standing is the examination of patient photographs. Patients should be asked to bring in old photos. Those with long-standing vertical deviations will reveal head tilts.

Measure vertical fusional ranges and examine old photographs to distinguish between acquired and congenital CN IV palsy.

In addition to vertical diplopia, patients with vertical deviations may complain of torsional diplopia. In this case, one image is tilted with respect to the other. Torsional diplopia is best measured by placing, in a trial frame, a white Maddox rod in front of one eye and a red Maddox rod placed in front of the other eye. The Maddox rods

Measure torsional diplopia with two Maddox rods.

are oriented vertically, so that the patient sees two straight lines, one above the other. If torsional diplopia is present, one line will appear tilted with respect to the other. The patient then rotates one or, if necessary, both Maddox rods until the lines appear parallel or superimposed. The amount of cyclotorsion in degrees is read from the trial frame.

Forced duction testing should be performed to determine whether any limitation in motility is due to a mechanical or nonmechanical, usually neurogenic etiology. This may be performed by way of two methods. After topical anesthesia is applied, forceps are used to grasp the conjunctiva and Tenon's fascia at the insertion of the muscle being tested. This is approximately 5 mm posterior to the

Perform forced duction test.

limbus. The patient is told to look in the direction of the restriction as the globe is pulled in this direction by the forceps. Alternatively, a cotton tip applicator placed just behind the limbus is used to push the eye in the direction of restriction. If the eye fails to move in this direction, a mechanical restriction is present and the test is "positive."

Causes of mechanical restriction include thyroid disease, muscle entrapment, tumor, inflammation, such as orbital pseudotumor, and Brown's tendon sheath syndrome. Oculomotor limitations due to neurological conditions will result in a negative test. However, it should be noted that over time neuropathic conditions might lead to muscle contraction, resulting in a positive forced duction test.

Primary Actions—Examination of Patient with Diplopia

- Determine whether the diplopia is monocular or binocular
  - If monocular
    - Perform pinhole test to determine whether it is due to media opacities or cerebral causes
  - If binocular—perform binocular testing
    - Determine whether comitant or incomitant
    - Isolate affected muscle(s)
    - Measure deviation in cardinal positions of gaze
    - Ocular motilities
    - Cover test
    - Red lens or Maddox rod
    - Park's three-step test

WORKUP OF COMMON CONDITIONS ASSOCIATED WITH BINOCULAR DIPLOPIA

Isolated Cranial Nerve Palsy

Third Nerve Palsy

The oculomotor nerve innervates the levator palpebrae superioris, the superior, inferior, and medial rectus muscles, and the inferior oblique. In a *complete* CN III palsy, the eye is turned out and down, and ocular movement is limited in all fields of gaze except laterally. The lid is ptotic. In an *incomplete* palsy, there is some movement of the globe.

Third nerve palsies may be limited to the superior or inferior division of CN III. In superior division palsy, there is ptosis and inability to elevate the eye. In inferior division palsy, there is inability to depress or adduct the eye. As in any case of a patient presenting with cranial nerve palsy, the clinician should test all cranial nerves.

Determine whether the CN III palsy is complete or incomplete.

Third nerve palsies may or may not affect the pupillary response. The pupil may be normal (spared), partially dilated, and poorly reactive, or fully dilated and unreactive.

Evaluate pupillary response.

In adults, the most common causes of third nerve palsies are infarction to the nerve and compression of the nerve from aneurysm. The most common site of the aneurysm is the posterior communicating artery. Pupillary fibers run peripherally in the nerve, making them more vulnerable to compression. Ischemia results in damage to the inner part of the nerve, not affecting the pupil.

A complete third nerve palsy that spares the pupil is *most likely* due to ischemia. However, it is thought that in up to 15% of complete third nerve palsies due to aneurysm, the pupil is spared. In addition, pupil involvement may be delayed. Particularly in cases of incomplete palsies, patients may present initially with a normal pupil, with involvement taking several days to occur. Thus, patients presenting with pupil-sparing third nerve palsies should be seen daily for the first five days to observe for signs of pupil involvement.

The most common cause of pupil-sparing third nerve palsies in patients over 50 is ischemic microvascular disease, such as hypertension, diabetes, and atherosclerosis. A large number of other systemic diseases have been associated with third cranial nerve palsy, including giant cell arteritis, meningitis, collagen-vascular dis-

Initially follow pupil-sparing CN III palsies on daily basis.

Table 13–6 Major Causes of Isolated Third Nerve Palsy

Adults

- Infarction
  - Diabetes
  - Hypertension
  - Atherosclerosis
- Aneurysm
- Meningitis
- Cavernous sinus disease
- Herpes zoster
- Giant cell arteritis
- Collagen vascular disease
- AIDS
- Multiple sclerosis
- Tumor

Children

- Congenital
- Trauma
- Aneurysm
- Tumor
- Migraine

ease, AIDS, tumor, and herpes zoster (Table 13–6). Thus, patients without a known history of vascular disease should be worked up for other systemic conditions as necessary. Giant cell arteritis has also been implicated. Patients over the age of 55 should have an erythrocyte sedimentation rate and C-reactive protein test to evaluate for giant cell arteritis.

Rule out giant cell arteritis in patients over 55.

Patients presenting with pupil-involving third nerve palsies should be referred for an immediate MRI and MRA of the brain to rule out aneurysm or mass. MRI and MRA should also be performed on patients younger than age 50. A neuro-ophthalmological consult should be obtained.

Refer for neuro-ophthalmological consult for CN III palsies involving pupil and in patients < 50.

Fourth Nerve Palsy

The trochlear nerve innervates the superior oblique muscle, which is responsible for making the eye intort and look down. Patients will complain of ver-

Table 13–7 Major Causes of Isolated Fourth Nerve Palsy

- Trauma
- Congenital
- Infarction
  ○ Hypertension
  ○ Diabetes
  ○ Atherosclerosis
- Idiopathic
- Multiple sclerosis

tical diplopia that is worse when looking to the side opposite the involved eye. In addition, one image may appear tilted.

In the case of left fourth nerve palsy, the patient tends to present with head tilt toward the right to compensate for intorsion weakness and chin directed downward to compensate for difficulty in moving the eye downward. Evaluation of patients with suspected fourth nerve palsies includes the Park's three-step test described above.

Perform Park's three-step test in cases of suspected CN IV palsy.

The most common causes of isolated fourth nerve palsy are trauma, ischemia, and a decompensation of a congenital phoria (Table 13–7). Trauma occurs bilaterally in approximately 30% of cases. A frequent source is whiplash from motor vehicle accidents. The source of the lesion is thought to be a contusion to nerve fibers in the anterior medullary velum.

Refer for neuro-ophthalmological consult patients who are younger or those without trauma or vascular risk factors.

Patients with congenital fourth nerve palsies will have increased fusional ranges. In addition, head tilt may be apparent from old photographs. In the case of acquired fourth nerve palsies, younger patients and patients with no history of vasculopathic risk factors or trauma should be referred for an MRI of the brain. Comanage with a neuro-ophthalmologist.

Sixth Nerve Palsy

The abducens nerve innervates the lateral rectus muscle, which causes the eye to turn out. Thus, patients with sixth nerve palsies will complain of horizontal diplopia, worse at distance than near, and worse in lateral gaze of the eye affected.

The most common cause of sixth nerve palsy in adults is infarction due

Table 13-8 Major Causes of Isolated
Sixth Nerve Palsy

Adults

- Infarction
  - ○ Diabetes
  - ○ Hypertension
  - ○ Atherosclerosis
- Congenital
- Trauma
- Metastatic disease
- Increased intracranial pressure
- Following spinal puncture
- Sarcoidosis
- Giant cell arteritis
- Cavernous sinus disease
- Stroke

Children

- Following viral illness
- Trauma
- Neoplasm (especially pontine glioma)
- Gradenigo's syndrome

to vascular diseases such as diabetes and hypertension (Table 13–8). Metastatic disease from breast or prostate cancer has also been implicated in patients with sixth nerve palsies. In children, sixth nerve palsies occur more frequently in the aftermath of viruses, trauma, and brainstem gliomas.

Workup for adults younger than 50 includes referral for MRI of the brain. Patients over 50 with known history of vasculopathic risk factors and no signs of giant cell arteritis may be monitored. In patients with a history of cancer a consult with the treating physician is indicated to rule out metastasis. Children without a recent history of viral illness should undergo MRI.

> *Refer for neuro-ophthalmological consult patients who are younger or without vascular risk factors.*

Myasthenia Gravis

This disease is characterized by a reduction in acetylcholine (Ach) receptors due to the presence of antibodies to those receptors. Neuromuscular transmission is impaired, especially during sustained activity when Ach is already reduced. Ptosis and variable extraocular muscle dysfunction are the hallmarks of this disease. The levator palpebrae superioris, extraocular muscles, and orbicularis oculi are affected, in addition to the muscles of facial expression, mastication, and proximal limb. Pupillary reactions are normal in the disease.

In evaluating for myasthenia, note any fluctuation in symptoms.

Myasthenia is typically bilateral, though it may present as unilateral early in the disease. It may or may not be associated with extraocular involvement. Ptosis and extraocular muscle function fluctuate and worsen with activity and late in the day.

A number of tests may be used in confirming the diagnosis of myasthenia gravis. The *sleep test* is a moderately sensitive test that takes advantage of the fact that ptosis and ocular motility improve after rest. The lid positions and extraocular motilities are observed before and after 30 to 45 minutes of patient rest. Any improvement is supportive of the diagnosis.

Cooling of the lids also improves neuromuscular transmission and reduces weakness. In the *ice test*, after the size of both palpe-

---
Evaluate extraocular muscle and lid function with the sleep test and the ice test.

---

bral apertures is measured, a surgical glove containing ice is applied to the more ptotic lid for two minutes. The other eye serves as a comparison. The size of the apertures is then compared. If there is a widening of the palpebral aperture in the eye the ice was applied to, then the test is positive. This will not be the case in ptosis of other origins. The ice test is highly sensitive and specific.

The patient's lid position may be measured before and after a minute of sustained upgaze. This will serve to fatigue the levator muscle. A worsening of ptosis is suggestive of myasthenia. Tensilon (edrophonium chloride) is an anticholinesterase that competes with Ach for acetyl-

---
Consider referral for Tensilon test.

---

cholinesterase, increasing the volume and time of Ach in the synapse. An intravenous injection of Tensilon will result in temporary lifting of the upper lid and improvement in ocular alignment in patients with myasthenia. However, paradoxical responses have been known to occur, which result in worsening of alignment. A positive test is strongly suggestive of myasthenia. A negative test does not necessarily rule it out.

Order Ach receptor antibody and thyroid function tests.

Initial workup of patients with suspected myasthenia includes the ordering of Ach receptor antibodies and thyroid function tests. A positive diagnosis necessitates referral to a neurologist for management.

Thyroid Ophthalmopathy (Graves' disease)

Graves' disease is an autoimmune disorder characterized by antibodies against the thyroid TSH receptor. The thyroid gland is continuously stimulated to produce and secrete hormones T_3 and T_4. Elevated levels are usually found in the serum. Ocular findings may precede positive laboratory results, however, so that testing may reveal the patient's state to be hyperthyroid, euthyroid, or hypothyroid. Thus, the diagnosis of Graves' disease is a clinical one.

Lid retraction is the most frequently occurring abnormality. Patients with Graves' disease have an increased likelihood of having myasthenia gravis, so that lid retraction may be masked by ptosis. In addition, lid retraction may be asymmetrical, so it may be difficult to determine which eye is abnormal. The examiner must determine whether there is an elevated lid in one eye or a ptotic lid in the other eye. Other lid abnormalities found in Graves' disease include lid lag in downward gaze, unilateral or bilateral proptosis, and lid edema.

Observe for lid retraction, lid lag, lid edema, and proptosis.

Extraocular muscle dysfunction leading to diplopia may occur in Graves' disease as a result of an extraocular muscle inflammation and infiltration. The primary muscles affected are the medial rectus and inferior rectus. The limitation is in the field of gaze opposite the muscle affected. Therefore, restriction is most likely to be found in elevation and abduction. A positive forced duction test will differentiate an abduction restriction due to Graves' disease from a sixth nerve palsy.

In cases of extraocular muscle restriction, perform forced duction test.

Other ocular manifestations of Graves' disease include conjunctival hyperemia in the areas overlying insertion of the horizontal rectus muscles, dry eye and superficial punctate keratitis due to exposure keratopathy, and optic nerve compression from thickened extraocular muscles.

Observe for signs of anterior segment inflammation and compressive optic neuropathy.

Workup of patients with Graves' disease includes thyroid function tests (T_4, T_3), thyroid-stimulating hormone (TSH), and CT scan of the orbits. The patient should be referred to an endocrinologist for management.

Comanage with endocrinologist.

MANAGEMENT

Management of patient diplopia in the emergency setting involves taking immediate action to eliminate the diplopia. Management is not necessarily geared toward establishing a permanent solution, but toward relieving disturbing patient symptoms as soon as possible.

In the case of monocular diplopia caused by media opacity such as a cataract, constricting the pupil with a miotic such as pilocarpine is often helpful. The clinician should use the smallest amount necessary to relieve the diplopia, starting with a 0.5% solution. An opaque tinted contact lens, with a clear pupillary zone, may also be used to treat monocular diplopia due to cataract or iris abnormalities. Other sources of monocular diplopia (e.g., kerataconus, astigmatism) need to be managed based upon the condition.

Reduce size of pupil pharmacologically or with contact lens.

To eliminate binocular diplopia, the central image must be blocked from one eye when the eye looks in the direction of gaze that elicits the diplopia. It is generally not necessary or advisable to occlude the eye entirely. All binocular vision need not be disrupted. Parts of the visual field may usually be left intact without the patient experiencing diplopia.

Semitransparent tape over the paretic eye of the patient's spectacles is often sufficient to eliminate the diplopia. If both eyes are paretic, then the tape should be placed over the eye with the least range of movement. If the patient does not have spectacles, then a pair of plano spectacles can be created. The tape need not cover the entire lens, but, rather, should be placed over those parts of the lens necessary to eliminate the diplopia.

Partially tape the spectacle over one eye to relieve the diplopia.

For example, in the case of a sixth nerve palsy, in which the patient experiences diplopia at distance, and not at near, tape should be placed over the central part of the lens, but not the lower part. This will enable the patient to utilize the lower part of the lens for reading. If the diplopia is in left gaze, then tape should be placed over the left portion of the lens.

Fresnel prism placed over the patient's spectacles may also be used to provide fusion in emergency situations. It should be remembered that the greater the amount of prism prescribed, the greater the degradation of the image. Therefore, the minimum amount necessary to relieve patient symptoms should be prescribed. This is usually in the range of one-half to three-quarters of the angle of deviation.

The intended prism prescription should first be placed into a trial frame and the patient should walk around with it for a time. The prism should be placed only over the paretic eye. For patients with oblique diplopia, nomograms are available, which will indicate the magnitude and direction of the prism based on the amount of horizontal and vertical diplopia measured separately.

Apply Fresnel prism on the spectacle over the paretic eye.

Options such as ground-in prism, botulinum toxin injections, and muscle surgery are available for long-standing diplopia. These interventions are used after the emergent situation. A course of vision therapy may also be employed to treat comitant deviations such as convergence insufficiency, strabismus, and decompensated phoria.

Initiate long-term strategies to alleviate diplopia depending upon etiology.

Primary Actions—Management of Patient with Diplopia

- If monocular
  - ○ Consider miotic, such as pilocarpine
  - ○ Opaque contact lens with clear pupil area
- If binocular
  - ○ Semitransparent tape over spectacles of paretic eye
    - ■ Limit position of tape to area of lens that eliminates diplopia
  - ○ Fresnel prism over spectacles of paretic eye
    - ■ Employ just enough to provide fusion
    - ■ Cut to fit part of lens depending on diplopic field of gaze
  - ○ Long-term management plan includes ground-in prism, surgery, and vision therapy

Chapter 14

Red Eye

"Doctor, my eye has become red!"

SCOPE OF THE PROBLEM

The red eye is a unique type of ocular emergency in a number of ways. Few ocular problems are associated with as many causes as the red eye. Red eyes are very common and may be manifestations of a wide variety of ocular and systemic conditions. Red eyes may be benign or may be a sight-threatening emergencies.

The fact that red eyes occur so frequently may not alert the patient or doctor to the severity of the condition. Patients may misinterpret the nature of the condition. They may attribute hyperemia to "pinkeye" and delay seeking medical attention. Their first action may be to use ocular vasoconstrictors, which mask signs of injection. Additionally, they may employ antibiotic drops given for a previous infection, or drops prescribed for another person.

HISTORY

Because the red eye has so many origins, patient history is crucial. It is often the most important piece of information the doctor will use. Knowing when the problem started is important in making the diagnosis; it should be kept in mind that patients may present for examination days or weeks after the onset of symptoms.

The following is a list of questions the examiner may use in taking a case history. Different questions will be emphasized depending upon the specific nature of the case (Table 14–1).

What is the *temporal and environmental context* in which the symptoms

Table 14–1   Outline of Questions for Red Eye Patient

- Time
    - Time of origin
    - Onset
        - Gradual
        - Sudden
    - Episodic or constant
    - Variability with time of day
- Environment
    - Locations—e.g., indoors, outdoors, dry
    - Exposure to toxic or chemical substances
    - Exposure to household products—soaps, detergents, hair sprays
    - Allergies
        - Airborne
        - Animal
        - Topical medications
    - Contact with other individuals with red eye
    - Potentially infectious environments—swimming pools, hot tubs, saunas
- Appearance of eye
    - Unilateral or bilateral
    - Location of injection
    - Periocular involvement
- Accompanying symptoms
    - Itching
    - Pain
        - Type and location of pain
    - Foreign body sensation
    - Photophobia
    - Discharge
        - Clear
        - Mucoid
        - Purulent
- Actions taken by patient
    - Treatment of condition to date
    - Use of eyedrops or ointments
    - Rubbing or manipulating the eye
- Ocular history
    - Previous episodes
    - History of surgery
    - Use of eye drops
    - Contact lens wearer
        - Type of lenses
        - Solutions
        - Time last worn
        - Typical wearing schedule
- Medical history

occurred? When was the red eye first noticed? Is
the problem of gradual or sudden onset? Is the
redness worse in any particular conditions, loca-
tions, or at any time of day? Are the lids "stuck
together" in the morning? Was the patient exposed to any chemical? Was the patient using any
new makeup, hair sprays, or detergents? Are there
any allergies, such as to animals or airborne sub-

*Ask about time and place
of symptoms.*

*Ask about appearance of
red eye.*

stances? Has the patient come into contact with anyone else who has recently
experienced a red eye? Was the patient in any environment in which ocular
infection may have been transmitted, such as a sauna or hot tub? Did the patient get a foreign substance in the eye? (see Chapter 11).

What is the *appearance* of the red eye? Is the injection unilateral or bilateral? The patient should be asked to describe the appearance of the eye
from the outset. Is the injection limited to any part of the eye, or does the
eye appear diffusely red? Did the patient note any lid or periocular involvement?

What are the *symptoms* associated with the red
eye? Does the eye itch? Does the patient experience
a foreign body sensation? Is the eye painful? "Superficial" pain may point in the direction of ocular surface disease, while "deep" pain and photo-

*Ask about symptoms that
accompany red eye.*

phobia are suggestive of intraocular inflammation, such as uveitis. However,
patients often have difficulty distinguishing between superficial and deep pain,
so the question may be of limited diagnostic value.

Is there a discharge present? Is it clear, mucoid, or purulent? Type of discharge reported, though suggestive of etiology, should also be interpreted with
caution. Patient descriptions are variable. For example, it is not unusual for a
patient with a dry eye resulting from an aqueous deficiency to complain of
"crusting" around the lids. It should not be misinterpreted as a mucoid discharge associated with an allergy, instead of due to reflex tearing and destabil-
ization of the tear film from a dry eye.

The actions taken by the patient should be asked. Did the patient flush the
eye, or use any eyedrops or ointments? Did the pa-
tient rub the eye, which may have resulted in increased injection, swelling, or corneal abrasion?
Has the patient been treated by another practitioner prior to presenting at your office?

*Ask about actions taken by
patient for red eye.*

The patient's *ocular history* should be investigated. Were there any pervi-
ous instances of red eyes? Were the symptoms similar? Was there a history of
surgery, which might suggest the possibility of a recurrent inflammation, dis-

ruption of an old wound, or delayed infection? Does the patient wear contact lenses? The wearing schedule—time last worn, average wearing time, overnight wear, brand, and solutions used—should be noted.

Take complete medical and ocular history.

There are a wide variety of systemic medical conditions that can be associated with the red eye. These include diseases of the skin and mucous membranes, as well as collagen vascular, cardio-vascular, neurological, immune, and metabolic diseases. Recent-onset illnesses, such as upper respiratory infections or flu-like symptoms, should also be noted.

Primary Actions—Case History on Patient with Red Eye

- Determine the temporal and environmental context of the red eye
- Obtain patient description of appearance of the red eye
- Identify the symptoms associated with the red eye
- Determine actions taken by patient in response to symptoms
- Obtain ocular history
  - Previous occurrences
  - Previous surgery
  - Contact lens wear
- Obtain medical history

EXAMINATION OF THE EMERGENCY RED EYE

The examination of the patient with a red eye is directed by the history. Based on the patient history, the clinician develops a clinical framework to account for the symptoms. Tables 14–2 and 14–3 provide such a framework to assist in diagnosis. The information provides a general classification of the more common causes of the acute red eye. Exceptions exist, and there is some over-lap among categories.

A detailed examination of the ocular structures should begin with a gross inspection of the patient's face and periocular area in bright illumination. The lids and area around the eyes should be inspected for injection, edema, scales, vesicles, and any skin lesions that may be present.

Examine face and periocular area, outside of instrument in bright light.

In performing biomicroscopy, lid examination should note any thickening, ectropion, entropion, trichiasis, flakes, mei-bomianitis, or madarosis. The tear film should be evaluated, noting whether it

Table 14-2 Signs and Symptoms Associated with Red Eye by Ocular Structure

- Pain
  - ○ Lid
    - ■ Cellulitis
  - ○ Conjunctiva/sclera
    - ■ Scleritis
    - ■ Hyperacute conjunctivitis
  - ○ Cornea
    - ■ Infectious ulcer
    - ■ Abrasion
  - ○ Uvea
    - ■ Anterior uveitis
  - ○ Global intraocular
    - ■ Endophthalmitis
  - ○ Orbital
    - ■ Orbital pseudotumor
    - ■ Specific orbital disease
  - ○ Cavernous sinus syndromes
- Photophobia
  - ○ Keratitis
  - ○ Uveitis
- Itching
  - ○ Contact dermatitis
  - ○ Allergic conjunctivitis (various forms)
- Foreign body sensation
  - ○ Ocular surface disease
- Discharge—associated with type of conjunctivitis
  - ○ Purulent
    - ■ Bacterial
    - ■ Hyperacute (*Neisseria gonorrhoeae, Neisseria meningitidis*)
    - ■ Fungal
  - ○ Mucopurulent
    - ■ Herpes simplex
    - ■ Herpes zoster
    - ■ Canaliculitis
    - ■ Dacryocystitis
    - ■ *Chlamydial* infection
  - ○ Mucoid/serous
    - ■ Herpes simplex
    - ■ Herpes zoster
    - ■ Rosacea
    - ■ EKC   *(continued)*

Table 14–2 *(continued)*

- ■ Pharyngoconjunctival fever
- ■ Allergic
- • Ocular motility restriction/proptosis
  - ○ Positive forced duction test
    - ■ Orbital inflammatory disease
    - ■ Graves' orbitopathy
  - ○ Negative forced duction test
    - ■ Cavernous sinus syndromes

Table 14–3   Red Eye Diagnoses by Primary Location of Inflammation

- • Lids
  - ○ Hordeolum
  - ○ Rosacea
  - ○ Contact dermatitis
  - ○ Cellulitis
- • Lacrimal system
  - ○ Dachryocystitis
  - ○ Canaliculitis
  - ○ Dacryoadenitis
- • Conjunctiva
  - ○ Diffuse
    - ■ Conjunctivitis (various forms)
    - ■ Keratitis
    - ■ Uveitis
    - ■ Endophthalmitis
    - ■ Infectious keratitis
    - ■ Orbital inflammatory disease
  - ○ Local
    - ■ Contact lens–associated red eye
    - ■ Superior limbal keratitis
    - ■ Scleritis
    - ■ Episcleritis
    - ■ Angular blepharitis
    - ■ Thyroid orbitopathy
- • Sclera
  - ○ Episcleritis—superficial vessels
  - ○ Scleritis—deeper vessels

is oily or scant. If inflammation of the lacrimal draining system is suspected, the medial canthal area should be carefully examined for signs of injection, swelling, or regurgitation of fluid.

Perform biomicroscopy to evaluate entire anterior segment.

The conjunctiva should be examined for papillae, follicles, hyperemia, and edema. Papillae tend to occur as polygonal clusters, and have a central vascular core. Follicles appear discrete, round, typically located inferiorly, and contain a vascular network around the edges of the follicle. The location of the hyperemia should be noted and whether it is focal or diffuse. Engorged vessels should be noted as to whether they are superficial or deep.

Each layer of the cornea should be evaluated. The epithelium should be examined for signs of superficial punctate keratitis (SPK). The stroma should be examined for infiltrates and signs of edema. In conditions such as iritis, cells may appear on the endothelium. The anterior chamber should be examined for signs of inflammation including cells, flare, and hypopyon. The iris should be evaluated for abnormalities such as neovascularization, and areas of atrophy. The lens should be evaluated for any signs of inflammatory material and posterior synechiae.

In evaluating the posterior segment, the clinician should examine the vitreous for cells, which may be indicative of endophthalmitis. The optic disc should be evaluated for edema, hyperemia, or hemorrhage, which may indicate orbital inflam-

Perform dilated fundus exam. Note any vitreoretinal inflammation.

matory disease. Retinal examination may show signs of posterior uveitis including retinal infiltrates or vasculitis.

External examination includes evaluation of extraocular muscles, pupils, and visual fields. Limitation of eye movements or proptosis is indicative of orbital disease. A dilated pupil is found in the case of acute angle closure glaucoma. Miosis is often seen in acute anterior

Evaluate motilities, pupils, and visual fields.

uveitis. Retinal or visual pathway defects may be revealed by confrontation visual fields.

Primary Actions—Examination of Patient with Emergency Red Eye

- Evaluate ocular structures, with assessment guided by case history
  - ○ Perform gross evaluation of face and periocular area
  - ○ Perform biomicroscopy, noting characteristic signs of ocular inflammation

○ Perform dilated fundus exam, noting any posterior segment causes of red eye
○ Perform external tests—motilities, pupils, and gross visual field evaluation

EMERGENCY RED EYE—ASSESSMENT AND MANAGEMENT

Disorders of the Lids and Lacrimal System

Preseptal cellulitis is an inflammation of the skin and subcutaneous tissue around the eye, anterior to the orbital septum. It presents with pain, diffuse swelling, warmth, and tenderness of one or both lids. There is accompanying conjunctival hyperemia, and little corneal involvement. The primary causes are infection from surrounding tissue, such as internal hordeolum, sinusitis, and dacryocystitis, or upper respiratory infection. *Staphylococcus* and *Streptococcus* are the most common etiologies, with *Hemophilus influenzae* common in children.

Patients with preseptal cellulitis should be placed on oral antibiotics for 10 days. Options include:

- Adults
  ○ Augmentin (amoxicillin/clavulanate), 500 mg, q8h
  ○ Keflex (cephalexin), 250 mg, q6h
  ○ Erythromycin, 250 mg, q6h
- In children over age five
  ○ Augmentin, 20–40 mg/kg/day in divided doses
  ○ Erythromycin, 30–50 mg/kg/day in divided doses

Manage preseptal cellulitis with oral antibiotics and warm soaks.

The patient should apply warm soaks to the eyelids three to four times a day. An antibiotic ointment may also be used. Consider hospitalization for children under age five and more severe cases.

A potential complication of preseptal cellulitis is expansion of infection beyond the orbital septum, resulting in orbital cellulitis.

Orbital cellulitis is an inflammation of the soft tissue of the orbit posterior to the orbital septum. It represents a much more serious disease than preseptal cellulitis, since it may lead to infection beyond the orbit. The disease may spread to the dural sinus, cavernous sinus, or meninges. Distinguishing preseptal from orbital cellulitis is critical. The former can be managed in the doctor's office, while the latter requires hospitalization.

Ocular signs found in orbital, but not presep-tal, cellulitis include proptosis, ocular motility re-strictions, and increased pain. Additionally, sys-temic symptoms are present, such as fever, nausea, and lethargy. Vision may be reduced. The major etiology is sinusitis, particularly in children. Other

Differentiate orbital from preseptal cellulitis by the presence of pain, proptosis, and motility restriction.

etiologies include infection from dental work, trauma, or ear infection. Patients with orbital cellulitis are treated with intra-venous antibiotics in the hospital. Referral should take place immediately, ow-ing to the severity of the condition.

Red eyes involving the lids of less severity include *internal and external* hordeolum. An *internal hordeolum* is an infection in a meibomian gland. An *external hordeolum* is an infection in a gland of Zeiss or Moll. The lesions pre-sent as a localized, tender nodular area. A con-comitant meibomianitis is usually seen. *Staphylo-coccus aureus* is the major infectious culprit. Management involves hot soaks several times a day. Topical antibiotic or combination steroid/antibi-otic medications are sometimes given to reduce

Manage hordeolum with hot soaks and, if needed, topical medications.

bacterial load or inflammation. Absent preseptal cellulitis, it is not necessary to place the patient on an oral antibiotic at the initial presentation.

Rosacea is a dermatitis associated with ocular complications such as ble-pharitis, meibomianitis, and hordeolum. It is usually noted in patients between the ages of 30 and 50. Signs include lid thickening, stasis of meibomian gland secretion, foamy tear film, and dilated conjunctival vessels. There is a flushed facial appearance, accompanied by rhinophyma, or hypertrophy of the nose, with sebaceous gland hyperplasia, and telangiectatic vessels. Corneal involve-ment presents as a superficial punctate keratitis (SPK), neovascularization, and scarring, particularly in the inferior region.

Treatment for rosacea consists of lid hygiene (warm soaks and cleansing), as well as application of antibiotic or antibiotic/steroid combination ointment to lids. Oral medications are used to en-hance meibomian gland secretions: tetracycline,

Manage rosacea with lid hygiene and tetracycline-family medications.

250 mg four times a day, or doxycycline, which is better tolerated, 100 mg bid. The medications should be used for one month, and then reduced by half if improvement is noted.

Contact dermatitis is another source of hyperemia to the periocular area. It is a type IV allergic reaction (involving thymus-derived lymphocytes), or de-layed hypersensitivity. It can take days to years to develop. It presents as peri-ocular eczema, with red, flaky, or scaly skin. Etiologies include eyedrops, ointments, or cosmetics. Though the eye itself is usually quiet, there may be conjunctival hyperemia and secondary infection.

Treatment includes avoidance of the offending agent and use of cool compresses. A topical steroid cream may be used, such as hydrocortisone, 1%, or dexamethasone, 0.05%, but caution must be used due to the possibility of creating a secondary infection. Additionally, the patient should be cautioned against getting the medication in the eyes when a nonophthalmic preparation is used.

Manage contact dermatitis by cool compresses, topical steroid cream, and avoidance of offending agent.

Acute *dacryocystitis* is an inflammation of the lacrimal sac. It is caused by stasis in the lacrimal drainage system resulting in infection. It can occur in infancy from congenital nasolacrimal duct obstruction. There is localized inflammation, pain, and edema, in the lower nasal canthal area. The lacrimal area is elevated. Pressing on the area results in a purulent discharge from the punctum. Patients complain of epiphora. Etiologies include *Staphylococcus aureus* and beta-hemolytic *Streptococcus*.

Treat dacryocystitis with warm soaks and oral antibiotics.

Initial management includes warm soaks with massage and topical antibiotic drops for congenital and acquired forms. For adults an oral antibiotic should be prescribed. Options include augmentin, 500 mg q8h, or keflex, 500 mg q6h. Nasolacrimal probing should not be performed on the eye during the acute stage.

Canaliculitis presents as hyperemia and pouting of the punctum. There is less swelling than in dacryocystitis and inflammation is limited to the area of the superior or inferior punctum. Symptoms are more chronic than acute. A purulent discharge may be expressed. The most common cause is *Actinomyces israelii*, a gram-positive bacterium that lodges in the canaliculus.

Comanage cases of canaliculitis with oculoplastic specialist.

Management involves culturing and staining of the punctal discharge. The primary treatment is removal of exudative or granular matter from the canaliculi, followed by irrigation with penicillin G solution. An oculoplastic specialist may perform this.

Note S shape and inflammation of temporal superior lid in dacryoadenitis.

Dacryoadenitis, or inflammation of the lacrimal gland, may present in acute or chronic forms. It may affect the palpebral lobe, orbital lobe, or both. The acute form is caused by a systemic bacterial or viral (e.g., mumps, mononucleosis) infection. The chronic form is often caused by a granulomatous disease, autoimmune disorder, or mass. In both forms there is inflammation of the temporal aspect of the superior lid, which assumes an S-shape configuration. The acute form is accompanied by more severe symptoms. The chronic form presents with a palpable mass in the superior temporal lid area. Proptosis and extraocular muscle restriction may occur in either form.

Management should be coordinated with the patient's primary care physician. Systemic workup should be performed to determine etiology. Laboratory testing should be performed on any discharge. Infectious causes should be ruled out. If a mass is suspected, a CT scan of the orbits and brain should be performed. Treatment depends upon etiology, and includes systemic medications.

> *Rule out granulomatous, autoimmune diseases, and masses in dacryoadenitis.*

Disorders of the Sclera and Conjunctiva

Episcleritis (Figure 14–1) is an inflammation of the superficial episcleral vessels. It is sectoral, usually appearing in the three or nine o'clock position. A nodule may be seen in the area. The patient may be asymptomatic or complain of mild irritation. The engorged vessels blanch with 2.5% phenylephrine. There may be an accompanying mild anterior uveitis. The disease is usually self-lim-

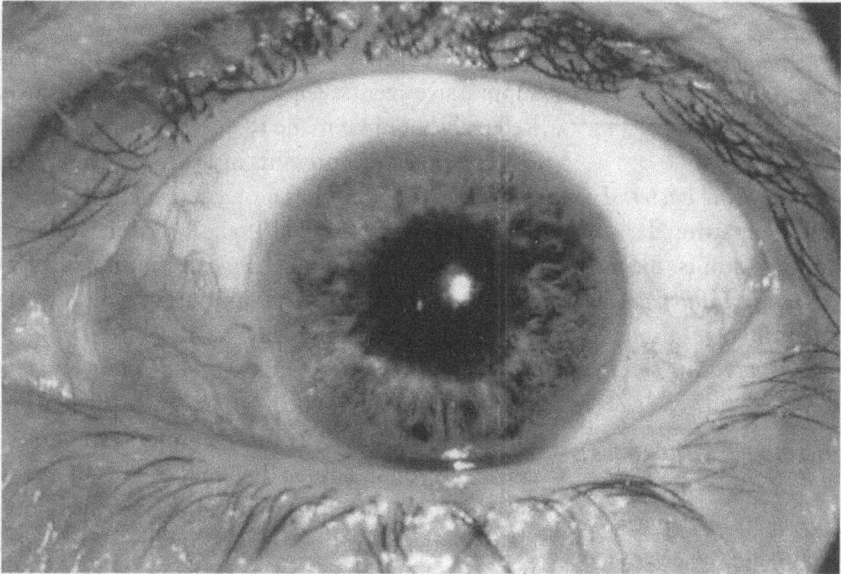

Figure 14–1. Episcleritis.

iting, lasting for 5 to 10 days, though it can last for months. In approximately 30% of cases, it is associated with a systemic disease. These include collagen vascular disease and infectious diseases such as syphilis and tuberculosis.

> Manage episcleritis with topical anti-inflammatory drops and oral NSAIDs in more severe cases.

Assuming there is not a significant medical history, systemic workup is not needed in first-time cases. Management options are various, depending on the signs and symptoms. They include artificial tears, vasoconstrictors, mild steroid drops, and oral or topical nonsteroidal anti-inflammatory (NSAID) medication.

Scleritis is a much more serious condition than episcleritis. In one-third of cases it is bilateral, usually occurring in women from the fourth to sixth decade of life. Symptoms include significant pain, photophobia, and tearing. There is dilation of deeper scleral vessels, giving the vessels a bluish color. These vessels do not blanch with 2.5% phenylephrine. There may be scleral edema, or scleral thinning, revealing visibility of the darker choroid beneath. This thinning should be distinguished from that seen in normal aging, which is usually symmetrical.

> Differentiate scleritis from episcleritis by presence of pain, ocular appearance, and association with systemic disease.

Over 50% of patients with scleritis have accompanying systemic disease, most commonly connective tissue disease. Medical management involves oral steroids and immunosuppressive agents. Topical steroids are ineffective. Referral should be made to a rheumatologist.

> Comanage scleritis with rheumatologist.

Conjunctivitis presents in a variety of forms. In typical *acute bacterial conjunctivitis*, the patient has a mucopurulent discharge and lid matting. It is primarily unilateral, but is likely to become bilateral over time. In adults, the most common cause is *Staphylococcus*. In children it is *Hemophilus influenzae*. There may be marginal corneal infiltrates. Typical treatment involves use of antibiotic drops four times a day.

Hyperacute conjunctivitis is primarily due to *Neisseria gonorrhoea*, and less frequently *Neisseria meningitidis*. It is spread from infected genitalia. It is more common in adolescents and young adults, though it can occur at any age. It presents with a substantial purulent discharge, edema of lids and conjunctiva, and pain. Preauricular lymphadenopathy may be present. It can be unilateral or bilateral. Other signs include

> Hyperacute conjunctivitis is associated with severe injection, purulent discharge, and Neisseria gonorrhoea.

SPK, stromal infiltrates, and corneal ulcer. This is an ocular emergency that can result in corneal perforation. The disease also may appear in newborns as a result of maternal gonorrhea.

Laboratory testing, including Gram and Giemsa staining and culture with chocolate agar, should be performed. Infants should be hospitalized, as should patients with severe corneal involvement. Treatment consists of intramuscular injection of ceftriaxone, 125 mg in patients with no corneal involvement to 1 g in those with corneal involvement. Topical treatment includes antibiotic ointment with frequency based

> *Refer suspected cases of hyperacute conjunctivitis for laboratory testing and intravenous antibiotics.*

upon severity. The patient should be referred for treatment immediately as ocular damage can occur very quickly.

Chlamydial keratoconjunctivitis disease results from an intracellular parasite, presenting with characteristics of both bacterial and viral disease. It is caused by the same parasite as trachoma, which is found in developing nations in crowded areas with poor hygienic conditions.

Chlamydia infection presents with large follicles, greater inferiorly, diffuse SPK, and occasional subepithelial infiltrates and pannus. In the case of trachoma, the follicles are more prominent on the superior conjunctiva and superior pannus is common.

> *Note large inferior follicles, mucopurulent discharge, and history of urogenital infection in* Chlamydial *disease.*

In contrast to forms of viral conjunctivitis, *Chlamydia* infection is usually limited to one eye and exhibits a mucopurulent discharge. It is transmitted from eye to eye or hand to eye. Like *Neisseria gonorrhoea*, it may also be transferred from infected mothers to newborns, occurring most commonly in the first week of life. *Chlamydia* is the most common cause of ophthalmia neonatorum. In adults, there is a history of genital or urinary tract infection. It may be acute or subacute. It frequently presents as a lingering conjunctivitis that has been misdiagnosed and treated unsuccessfully in the past.

Conjunctival culturing and scrapings of the conjunctival epithelium with Giemsa or Wright stain may be used in diagnosis of *Chlamydia* infection. The patient should be treated with an oral antibiotic (Table 14–4). Treatment with topical antibiotic ointment is considered as an adjunct to oral medication.

> *Manage* Chlamydia *infection with laboratory testing and oral antibiotics.*

The tetracylines should not be used in children below age eight, pregnant women, or breast-feeding mothers.

Viral conjunctivitis exhibits a watery discharge, follicles on the inferior

Table 14–4 Treatment Options for Chlamydia in Adults

Oral antibiotics

- Azithromycin, 1 g (repeat one week later, if necessary)
- Tetracycline, 250–500 mg qid for 2 weeks
- Doxycycline, 100 mg bid for 2 weeks
- Erythromycin, 500 qid for 7 days

Supplementary topical antibiotic ointments

- Erythromycin bid-qid
- Tetracycline bid-qid

palpebral conjunctiva, and a tender preauricular lymph node. It usually begins in one eye and spreads to the other eye within a week. Corneal involvement may reveal superficial punctate keratitis and subepithelial infiltrates. Pseudomembranes may be present. A number of common acute forms of viral conjunctivitis exist, including epidemic keratoconjunctivitis (EKC), pharyngoconjunctival fever (PCF), and acute hemorrhagic conjunctivitis.

> In diagnosing viral conjunctivitis, look for follicles, SPK, SEIs, pseudomembranes, and flu-like symptoms.

Epidemic keratoconjunctivitis (Figure 14–2) presents with subepithelial infiltrates (SEIs) on the fourteenth to twentieth day of the disease. It is caused by an adenovirus, usually type 8 or 19. It is highly contagious, spreading from the respiratory tract to the eye, from hand to eye, or by contact with contaminated ophthalmic instruments. Treatment is supportive: cool compresses, artificial tears, and vasoconstrictors. Topical steroids will prolong the course of the disease, and should not be used unless vision is significantly compromised. Precautions against transmission of infection should be discussed with the patient.

> Manage viral conjunctivitis supportively with cool compresses, lubricants, and vasoconstrictors.

Pharyngoconjunctival fever manifests milder signs and symptoms than EKC. Subepithelial infiltrates may be present, but they are smaller than in the case of EKC. The disease is caused by an adenovirus, usually type 3 or 7. Patients have pharyngitis and fever. The disease is likely to be transmitted via swimming pools.

Acute hemorrhagic conjunctivitis is caused by an enterovirus, usually type 70. It is transmitted from hand to eye. The disease exists in epidemic forms in Asia, Africa, and the Americas. It may present with a serous or mucoid discharge. There are bilateral subconjunctival pinpoint hemorrhages on the up-

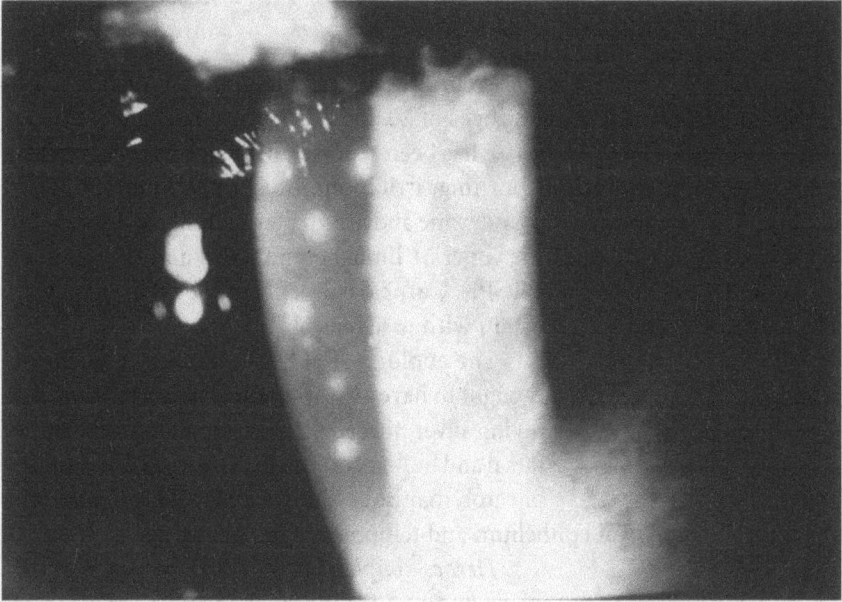

Figure 14–2. Subepithelial infiltrates in EKC.

per palpebral or bulbar conjunctiva, which take one to two weeks to resorb. Corneal signs include superficial punctate keratitis and subepithelial infiltrates. There may be a history of flu-like symptoms and enlarged preauricular nodes. The disease typically resolves by 10 days. Management is supportive, including artificial tears and vasoconstrictors.

Seasonal allergic conjunctivitis involves chemosis of the lids, in greater proportion than erythema. The hallmark symptom is itching. It presents bilaterally, with papillae found underneath the lid. A mucoid discharge is present. It may be treated with a wide variety of antiallergy drops including vasoconstrictors, antihistamines, mast cell stabilizers, and mild steroids.

Vernal conjunctivitis can be considered a variant of allergic conjunctivitis. The disease occurs in the spring and is found in increased incidence in young boys. In addition to the symptoms of seasonal allergic conjunctivitis, there may be corneal involvement. Horner-Trantas dots, or elevated areas of degenerated eosinophils, may be present in the limbal area or on the bulbar conjunctiva. There may also be a corneal shield ulcer, in the form of a gray infiltrate. Management involves topical steroids or mast cell stabilizers. If a shield ulcer is present, a topical antibiotic should be added.

> *Antihistamines, mast cell stabilizers, and mild steroids can be used to treat varieties of allergic conjunctivitis.*

CORNEAL DISORDERS

Superior limbic keratitis (SLK) is chronic, recurrent keratoconjunctivitis occurring in patients between the ages of 20 and 60. Seventy-five percent of patients are female. Thyroid disease has been reported in a large number of these patients. Symptoms include burning, irritation, foreign body sensation, and photophobia. Symptoms wax and wane and are greater than signs. There is hyperemia and thickening of the superior limbal conjunctiva and superior tarsus, as well as superior corneal SPK. Corneal filaments may be present as well. The cornea and conjunctiva stain with rose bengal.

Use silver nitrate solution to manage SLK.

The etiology of SLK is unknown, though it is thought to have an immunological association. Applying silver nitrate, 0.5–1%, solution to the upper tarsal and bulbar conjunctiva, using a cotton tip applicator, may be used to treat SLK. This removes the abnormal conjunctival epithelium and temporarily relieves symptoms.

Primary HSV usually resolves without treatment.

Herpes simplex virus (HSV) presents in primary and recurrent ocular forms. Primary HSV occurs in childhood. It presents as a unilateral blepharoconjunctivitis, with vesicular lesions on the lid, follicles, and sometimes keratitis. It resolves without treatment. Antibiotic ointments may be given two to four times a day.

Recurrent HSV usually presents as a unilateral red eye with mild to moderate symptoms, including foreign body sensation, tearing, and photophobia. Corneal epithelial disease is marked by the classic dendrite (Figure 14–3), which stains well with rose Bengal. Initially the cornea may exhibit only a superficial punctate keratitis. Cornea hypoesthesia is present. Recurrences are common, and episodes tend to worsen with recurrence.

Corneal defects in secondary HSV include unilateral dendrites, stromal scarring, and neurotrophic ulcer.

Corneal stromal disease occurs in 10–15% of cases with recurrent keratitis. Stromal scarring and disciform, necrotizing, or interstitial keratitis may occur. There may also be iritis and multifocal choroiditis.

Manage HSV epithelial disease with antiviral agents.

Following the epithelial disease a neurotrophic or metaherpetic ulcer may occur, without active stromal disease. The ulcer may be dendritic, round, or oval with sinuous or scalloped borders and rolled edges. Damage to corneal innervation results in the epithelial defect.

Management depends upon what part of the

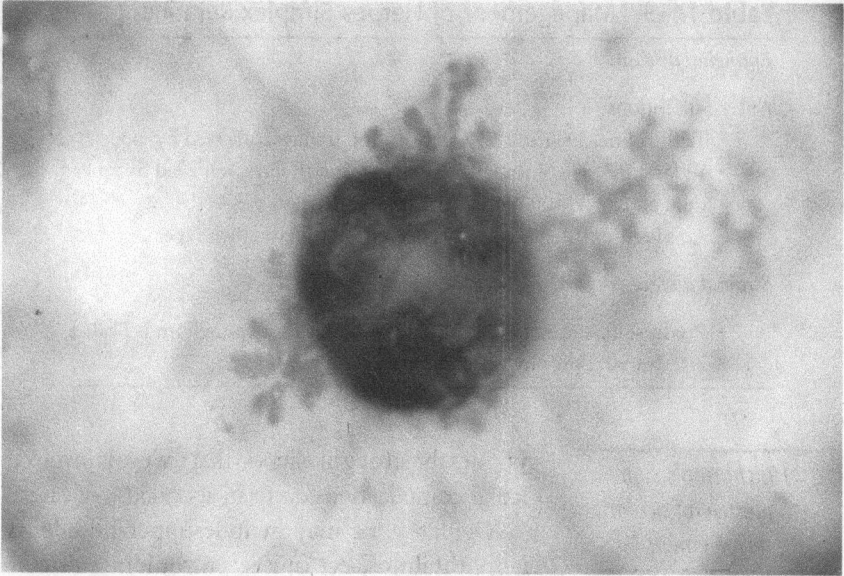

Figure 14–3. HSV dendritic keratitis.

eye is involved. (See Table 14–5.) For epithelial keratitis, a number of antiviral agents may be used. If stromal disease occurs, a topical steroid should be used once the epithelium has healed. The antiviral should be continued (a one-to-one basis with the steroid is usually sufficient) prophylactically to prevent epithelial disease from recurring. The drops may be used every one to four hours followed by taper.

> *Manage HSV stromal disease with antiviral agents and topical steroids.*

Herpes zoster virus (HZV) manifests signs following the dermatome of the first division of the fifth cranial nerve. There is reactivation of the HZV in the dorsal root ganglion or trigeminal ganglion. It has a tendency to occur in immunosuppressed individuals as well as in diseases such syphilis and tuberculosis, and trauma. The skin presents with an initial blushing, followed by appearance of papules, and then vesicles, which burst to form crusts. Later, white scars form in the area. The lesions are limited to one side of the face.

> *Observe for skin lesions following dermatome of CN VI.*

Symptoms include pain, tingling, and numbness in the affected area. The incidence of neuralgia, which may last six months or longer, increases with age of the patients. Hutchinson's sign, or the presence of a lesion at the tip of the nose,

Table 14–5   Management of Herpes Simplex Keratitis

Epithelial disease

Antiviral Options
- Trifluridine, 1% drops, 9X per day for 10 days, followed by taper
- Vidarabine, 3% ointment, 5X per day for 10 days, followed by taper
- Oral acyclovir, 400 mg, 5X per day for 10 days
- Acyclovir ointment, 3%, 5X per day for 10 days, then taper

Stromal disease

- Prednisolone acetate, 1%, every 1–4 hours after epithelium is healed
- Use antiviral prophylactically

Hutchinson's sign suggestive of ocular involvement.

Observe for pseudodendrites, stromal scarring, and uveitis.

indicates the strong likelihood that the eye is involved. Ocular complications occur in about 50% of cases.

Ocular signs may include upper lid edema, lagophthtalmos, ectropion, entropion, and conjunctival injection. The cornea is involved in about 40% of HZV cases. The most common corneal signs are "pseudodendrites" or SPK. Pseudodendrites are usually seen in the acute stage for four to six days. They usually resolve without treatment. Unlike those found in HSV, the dendrite has no terminal end bulbs. Stromal disease may present as a disciform (similar to HSV), necrotizing, or interstitial keratitis.

Uveitis is frequent in HZV. Single or multiple patches of sectoral iris pigment loss occur due to local vasculitis. In rare cases, patients can present with retinal vasculitis and optic neuritis. Systemic symptoms include headache, malaise, fever, and chills.

Treatment should be instituted as soon as possible to improve prognosis. Treatment should be initiated within the first three days, but may be given up to a week. An oral antiviral should be prescribed, for a course of 10 days (Table 14–6). Mild antibiotic ointments should be applied to skin lesions, along with cool compresses and mechanical cleansing. Corneal SPK or pseudodendrites may be treated with lubricants. Stromal keratitis should be treated with steroids, such as prednisolone acetate, 1%, q1h to q6h. Cycloplegia should be added in cases of anterior uveitis.

Manage HZV with oral antiviral agents.

Manage ocular involvement with lubricants, steroids, and cycloplegia.

For discussion of *corneal abrasion*, see Chapter 12.

Table 14–6 Management of Herpes Zoster

Oral antiviral for 10 days
- Options
    - Acyclovir, 800 mg, 5X/day.
    - Famciclovir, 500 mg tid
    - Valacyclovir, 1000 mg tid

SPK or pseudodendrites
- Ocular lubricants

Stromal disease
- Topical steroid, e.g., prednisolone acetate, 1%, q1h to q6h

Uveitis
- Topical steroid
- Cycloplegia

Bacterial corneal ulcer (Figure 14–4) is one of the most severe and painful ocular emergencies. It presents as a focal area of epithelial defect and underlying stromal infiltrate. Primary etiologies include *Staphylococcus aureus, Streptococcus pneumoniae, Pseudomonas aeruginosa, Hemophilus influenzae,* and *Moraxella.* The lesion is typically surrounded by stromal edema.

> *Look for excavated epithelial defect with underlying stromal infiltrate.*

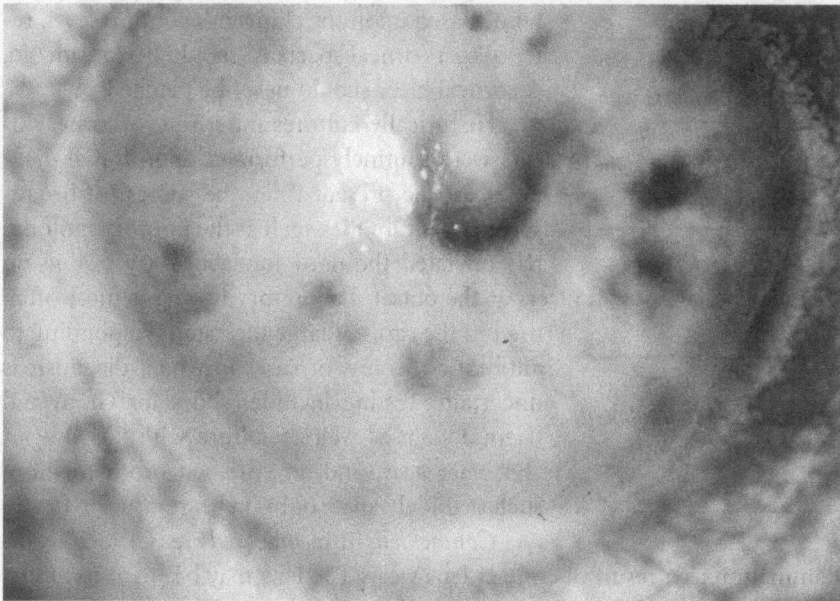

Figure 14–4. Bacterial corneal ulcer in a soft contact lens wearer.

An infectious corneal ulcer should be distinguished from a "sterile" corneal infiltrate. The sterile infiltrate is considered an inflammatory reaction to bacterial exotoxins. While the sterile infiltrate may have a small amount of overlying staining, the infectious ulcer has the appearance of an excavation into the cornea. Patients with corneal ulcers are more symptomatic than those with sterile infiltrates. They will report pain and photophobia. The presence of an anterior chamber reaction is much more likely in the case of an ulcer as well.

Distinguish ulcer from sterile infiltrate by presence of pain, photophobia, staining pattern, and uveitis.

Management of corneal ulcers is somewhat variable, depending on size and area of cornea involved. Typical therapy consists of a second generation fluoroquinolone, such as Ciprofloxacin or Ofloxacin drops, q15min for six hours, then every half-hour until the next day. Newer third and fourth generation fluoroquinolones have not been approved for corneal ulcers as of this writing. A topical ointment, such as polysporin two to four times a day, provides increased antibacterial coverage. Cycloplegia should also be initiated. The patient should be seen the next day.

Many ulcers can be managed with topical fluoroquinolone and antibiotic ointment.

Patients with large (>1.5 m in diameter) or vision-threatening ulcers should be given fortified tobramycin or gentamycin, 15 mg/mL every hour, alternating with fortified cefazolin, 50 mg/mL every hour. Based upon the clinician's comfort level, referral to a corneal specialist should be considered. A corneal ulcer should never be patched.

Manage large or vision-threatening ulcers with fortified antibiotics. Consider consult with corneal specialist.

Historically, cultures and smears of corneal ulcers were routinely performed upon initial diagnosis. At the present time, the success of broad-spectrum antibiotics such as the fluoroquinolones has obviated the need for laboratory testing on many bacterial corneal ulcers at the outset. Laboratory testing is most often used in the cases of large ulcers not responding to antibiotic therapy, or cases in which diagnosis is uncertain. Testing includes slides for Gram and Giemsa stain as well as culture with blood agar, chocolate agar, and an enriched broth medium such as thioglycolate or brain heart infusion broth.

Culture ulcers unresponsive to treatment or when diagnosis is uncertain.

Contact lens–associated red eye (CLARE) is inflammation as a result of contact lens wear. The lens may be worn too long, be too tight, or be laden with deposits. The patient may experience some pain, but not the severe pain associated with an infectious ulcer. Conjunctival injection is present, which is greater in the limbal area due to hypoxia. Corneal neovascularization may be seen. There may be small infiltrates, particularly in the peripheral cornea with pinpoint staining overlying the infiltrates. These infiltrates are differentiated from those of an infectious ulcer by their small size, lack of stromal excavation, limbal location, and absence of an anterior chamber reaction. Gram-negative bacteria on contact lenses have been found in cases of CLARE. This does not cause frank infection but creates an inflammatory response due to the release of bacterial endotoxins.

> *With CLARE, look for limbal injection and small limbal infiltrates.*

Management always includes discontinuation of lens wear. Antibiotic/steroid drop combinations are effective in reducing inflammation and treating any bacterial component that may be present.

Fungal keratitis is less common than that of bacterial and viral origin. There is a history of ocular exposure to plants or vegetative matter, often as a result of trauma. The most common causes are *Fusarium*, *Candida*, and *Aspergillus*. Infections tend to occur in tropical or subtropical climates. They are more likely to occur in individuals whose immune system is compromised, such as those with AIDS, or those being treated with chemotherapy or steroids. There is a slow, insidious onset, often over a period of weeks.

> *Note history of exposure to vegetable matter, insidious onset, and whether patient is immunocompromised.*

Fungal ulcers often appear as elevated grayish-white stromal infiltrates, with irregular feathery borders. The epithelium may or may not be intact. Smaller, infiltrative satellite lesions may occur away from the main lesion. The infection gradually progresses to invade the deeper cornea. The lesion may be surrounded by a ring infiltrate of white blood cells. Purulent discharge and hypopyon are often seen.

> *Look for stromal infiltrates with irregular borders.*

If a fungal infection is suspected, laboratory studies are needed. Corneal smears and cultures should be ordered. Stains to order include Giemsa, Gram, calcofluor white, and Gomori's methenamine silver. Culture media include Saboraud dextrose agar, and brain-heart infusion broth. It can take up to two weeks to confirm no growth, but 80% of fungal infections show growth within three days.

Prior to definitive diagnosis, potential cases of fungal keratitis are treated as of bacterial eti-

> *Order laboratory studies. Treat as bacterial until proven otherwise. Avoid steroids.*

Refer confirmed cases of fungal keratitis to corneal specialist.

ology. Cases of fungal keratitis are best managed by a corneal specialist. Any steroids the patient is taking should be discontinued. Antifungal medications are highly toxic, and exhibit limited corneal penetration and effectiveness. These include amphotericin B, natamycin, imidazole compounds, and fluctosine.

UVEITIS

Anterior uveitis, consisting of inflammation of the iris and ciliary body, is another source of acute red eye (Figure 14–5). There are a number of etiologies, the most common being idiopathic. (See Table 14–7.) Symptoms include ocular pain and, particularly, sensitivity to light. There will be a circumlimbal flush, and cells and flare in the anterior chamber. A miotic pupil and lower intraocular pressure in the involved eye are often seen. Posterior synechiae, fibrin on the lens, and "spillover" cells in the vitreous may be present in more severe cases.

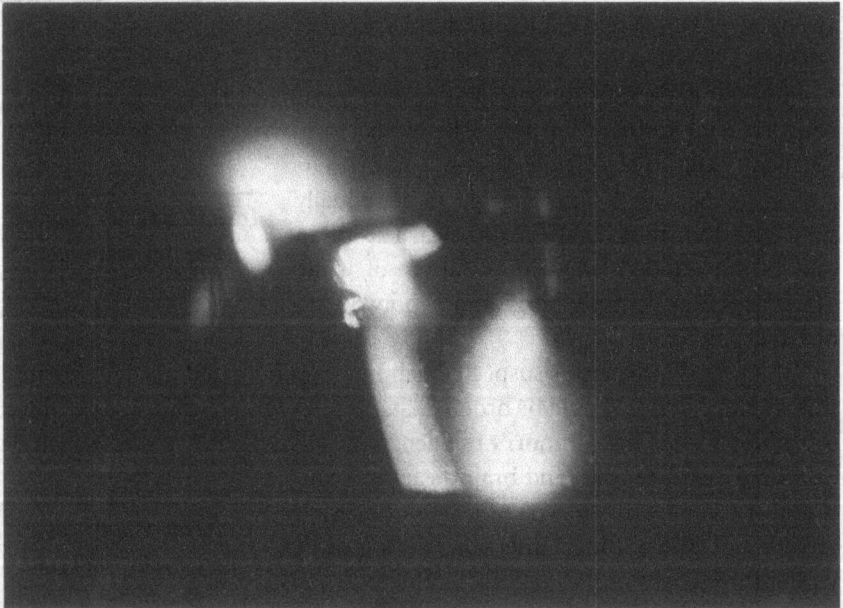

Figure 14–5. Acute, anterior, unilateral uveitis in an HLA-B27 positive male.

Table 14–7   Most Common Causes of Uveitis

Anterior
- Idiopathic
- HLA-B27 spondyloarthropathies
- Juvenile rheumatoid arthritis associated
- Herpes simplex/zoster
- Fuchs heterochromatic
- Intraocular lens related
- Sarcoidosis
- Traumatic

Intermediate
- Idiopathic
- Sarcoidosis
- Multiple sclerosis

Posterior
- Toxoplasmosis
- Retinal vasculitis
- Idiopathic
- Ocular histoplasmosis
- Toxocariasis
- Cytomegalovirus retinitis
- Serpiginous choroidopathy
- Acute multifocal placoid pigment epitheliopathy
- Necrotizing herpetic retinopathy
- Birdshot choroidopathy
- Sarcoidosis

Panuveitis
- Idiopathic
- Sarcoidosis
- Vogt-Koyanagi-Harada
- Multifocal choroiditis
- Behçet syndrome

Adapted from Basic and Clinical Science Course, Intraocular Inflammation and Uveitis, 2001, the Foundation of the American Academy of Ophthalmology.

Anterior uveitis can present in granulomatous and nongranulomatous forms. Large "mutton fat" keratic precipitates located on the corneal endothelium characterize the granulomatous form. It is often bilateral. Nongranulomatous forms present with fine keratic precipitates.

> *Observe for cells and flare, KPs, miosis, and reduced IOP.*

Patients with a first-time, unilateral, nongranulomatous condition do not

Evaluate for systemic disease as appropriate.

need to be worked up for systemic disease unless one is suspected. Patients with a granulomatous uveitis should be tested for sarcoidosis, syphilis, and tuberculosis.

Emergency management for anterior uveitis includes topical steroids and cycloplegia. Prednisolone acetate, 1%, is usually the drug of choice. It should be used more often during the first few days and then tapered. In more severe cases it may be used as often as every hour the first day. Cycloplegics should be used once to three times a day, depending upon presentation.

Dilate all patients with anterior uveitis. Manage with topical steroids and cycloplegics.

Cases of anterior uveitis may have signs of inflammation originating in the posterior segment or even the central nervous system. Therefore, it is important that every patient presenting with an anterior uveitis be dilated. Cases of posterior uveitis with "spillover" into the anterior segment may present with a red eye, creating a *panuveitis*. Vitritis, retinitis, choroiditis, or optic disc swelling may be found. Diseases such as lymphoma can originate in the eye or central nervous system. In addition to bilateral ocular inflammation, patients may experience neurological symptoms including confusion, weakness, and deterioration in mental functioning. Referral to the appropriate medical specialist should be initiated.

Observe for signs of panuveitis.

For discussion of acute angle-closure glaucoma, see Chapter 15.

ENDOPHTHALMITIS

Endophthalmitis is an infectious red eye involving both the anterior chamber and vitreous. It is a potentially sight-threatening emergency. There are several different kinds, including traumatic, postoperative, bleb-associated, and endogenous. (See Chapters 12 and 19.) Vision is decreased and the eye is highly inflamed and painful.

Note symptoms of a severely painful eye, with reduced vision.

Postoperative endophthalmitis may be acute or chronic. The acute form occurs within one to 14 days postsurgery. *Staphylococcus* is the primary etiology. There are fewer instances than in the past with the advent of small-incision cataract surgery. Infection can occur by contaminated instruments.

Chronic or delayed-onset postoperative endophthalmitis occurs four or more weeks after surgery. Symptoms are insidious, and may be dampened by postoperative antibiotic therapy. Fungi and *Propionobacterium acnes*, contained in the normal skin flora, are among the more likely causes. There is a persistent uveitis despite topical steroid therapy. Anterior chamber and vitreal tap are performed for diagnostic purposes. The patient is treated with intravitreal therapy. In the case of infections involving the lens implant, it may be necessary to remove infected material from the posterior capsular bag.

> *Consider the possibility of endophthalmitis in patients with persistent inflammation following surgery.*

Bleb-associated endophthalmitis should be distinguished from "blebitis." In the case of the latter, there is a low-grade inflammation of bleb, which appears thin and cystic. In the former, the bleb is infected, with vitritis and hypopyon present.

Endogenous endophthalmitis occurs from bloodborne spread of bacteria or fungi during generalized septicemia. Patients are chronically ill with diseases such as diabetes or renal failure. They may be immunosuppressed, or using intravenous drugs. The disease presents with a very

> *Refer cases of endophthalmitis to vitreo-retinal specialist.*

acute onset, reduced vision in each eye, hypopyon, and vitritis. Hospitalization is required, with the initiation of treatment following laboratory testing.

Endophthalmitis of any origin constitutes an emergency, which is generally not treated initially in the individual practitioner's office. Cases are usually managed by a vitreoretinal specialist. Hospitalization is typically required. (See Chapter 12.)

ORBITAL RED EYES

The clinical features differentiating orbital red eyes from those not involving the orbit are proptosis and/or ocular motility restriction. They may be broadly categorized as nonspecific or specific (Table 14–8).

> *Consider orbital involvement in cases with proptosis and EOM restriction.*

Orbital pseudotumor refers to orbital inflammation not caused by a specific disease. There is a positive forced duction test. The disease is marked by infiltrations of polymorphous inflammatory cells, rather than granulomas or masses, which

> *Order orbital imaging studies.*

Table 14–8   Red Eyes Involving the Orbit

Nonspecific (orbital pseudotumor)
- Apical
- Lacrimal
- Diffuse
- Anterior
- Myositic

Specific
- Infectious
  - ○ Orbital cellulitis
  - ○ Fungal infections
    - ■ Mucormycosis
    - ■ Aspergillosis
  - ○ Tuberculosis
  - ○ Syphilis
- Orbital vasculitis
  - ○ Wegener's granulomatosis
  - ○ Polyarteritis nodosa
- Granulomatous inflammations
  - ○ Sarcoidosis
  - ○ Orbital xanthogranulomas
- Tumors
- Graves' orbitopathy

have a more chronic presentation. It is idiopathic, typically unilateral, and rarely associated with systemic disease. Unlike in cases of orbital cellulitis, patients are afebrile.

There is an acute or subacute onset of a painful, edematous red eye. The disease is classified according to the primary orbital area of inflammation: anterior, apical, diffuse, lacrimal, or myositic (extraocular muscles). Uveitis, as well as optic disc edema, and retinal detachment may be found. An orbital CT scan should be ordered. Primary treatment is with systemic corticosteroids. Patients will require ophthalmological follow-up.

Orbital red eyes with specific etiologies are usually associated with infections, as in the case of orbital cellulitis (see above), or accompanied by systemic disease. The latter typically present with more chronic symptomatology.

RED EYES ASSOCIATED WITH DISORDERS POSTERIOR TO THE ORBIT

These are known as *cavernous sinus syndromes*. The cavernous sinuses are paired venous channels, located on either side of the sphenoid sinuses. Traveling through the cavernous sinus are cranial nerves three, four, and six, the ophthalmic and maxillary branch of cranial nerve five, and the internal carotid artery with its sympathetic plexus. Major characteristics of red eyes due to cavernous sinus syndromes include unilateral "deep," painful ophthalmoplegia and proptosis. The ophthalmoplegia may not be limited to one nerve. In contrast to red eyes due to orbital inflammations, there is typically a negative forced duction test and no resistance to retropulsion.

Look for painful ophthalmoplegia and proptosis.

Rule out specific (e.g., infectious) etiologies. Co-manage with physician.

Other distinguishing features include facial pain or anesthesia along the first or second branches of the fifth cranial nerve, ptosis, and miosis (Horner's syndrome). Fundus findings may be present in the form of optic disc edema and retinal hemorrhages. Diagnostic workup includes neuroimaging of the orbit and sellar regions. Table 14–9 lists etiologies of the cavernous sinus syndrome.

Differentiate from orbital pseudotumor by negative forced duction test, absence of resistance to retropulsion, and sympathetic and fifth nerve involvement.

The emergency care clinician needs to consider the possibility that the red eye may relate to disease in the orbit or cranium. The doctor needs to be aware

Table 14–9 Etiologies of Cavernous Sinus Syndrome

- Carotid-cavernous fistula
- Cavernous sinus tumor
- Cavernous sinus aneurism
- Cavernous sinus thrombosis
- Tolosa-Hunt syndrome (idiopathic)
- Metastatic lesions
- Primary brain tumors
- Herpes Zoster

> *Obtain neuro-ophthalmological consultation.*

of the constellation of signs and symptoms that differentiate these red eyes from others. Though the etiology usually cannot be identified at the initial visit, it is important that the patient be referred to the appropriate specialist. When cavernous sinus disease is suspected, the patient should be referred to a neuro-ophthalmologist.

Primary Actions—Assessment and Management of Patient with Red Eye

- Determine the cause(s) of the red eye
- Localize the primary origin of the inflammation
- Evaluate the urgency of the condition
- Provide medical treatment
- Order additional laboratory and imaging studies as needed
- Arrange consultation with other providers as appropriate

Chapter 15

Acute Eye Pain

"Doctor, when I woke up this morning my eye was killing me!"

SCOPE OF THE PROBLEM

The presence of pain in and around the eye can be due to relatively minor problems or may be an indicator of significant ocular pathology. Occasionally, pain centered on the eye is actually referred pain from elsewhere. Regardless of etiology, pain is significant to the patient and when a patient presents acutely because of it, the cause needs to be ascertained and treated and the pain alleviated.

The variety of causes of ocular pain will be discussed in this chapter with emphasis being placed on those that will cause a patient to present urgently.

HISTORY

As with all patient complaints, the onset, duration, frequency, severity, progression, and quality of the pain should be determined. Severity of the pain may not be a good indicator of the severity or location of the condition, however, as pain receptors are con-centrated in the anterior portion of the eye. Rela-tively minor injuries affecting anterior structures might be associated with severe pain whereas significant posterior inflammation can have little or no pain (Table 15–1). Pain can be referred to the ocular or periocular area from relatively distant sites, making localization difficult.

> *Ask about onset, duration, frequency, severity, progression, and quality of pain.*

Symptoms such as photophobia or reduced vision should be sought as

Table 15–1   Potential Causes of Acute Eye Pain

Dry eye and keratoconjunctivitis sicca
Blepharitis
   Meibomianitis
   Hordeola
   Marginal corneal infiltrates
   Peripheral corneal ulcers
Preseptal/orbital cellulitis
Dacryocystitis
Conjunctivitis
   Viral (EKC)
   Allergic
Episcleritis/pingueculitis
Scleritis
Corneal conditions
   Abrasion
   Erosion
   Ulceration
   Infiltration
Uveitis
   Acute, unilateral anterior
   Other—bilateral, posterior, chronic
Angle-closure glaucoma
Optic neuritis
Orbital disease
Parasellar disease
Posterior fossa disease
Sinus disease
Migraine

Ask about symptoms accompanying pain.

these may help determine the location and cause of the pain. The presence of photophobia increases the likelihood that the patient will have an inflammatory condition. Reduced vision implicates a problem affecting the visual axis or retina or optic nerve.

Dry eye syndrome is a very common problem in which the patient complains of a foreign body sensation. In almost all cases, patients with dry eye will not present with an acute complaint. However, an acute exacerbation of the condition because of environmental factors, associated ocular factors, or change in systemic health can occasionally cause the patient with dry eye to present with a more urgent complaint. Patients with severe dry eye (keratoconjunctivitis sicca) usually have an underlying autoimmune or connective tissue disorder. Acute symptomatology from the dry eye is often correlated with an increase in activity of their systemic disease. The optometrist should seek a history of

Ask about dry eye symptoms and associated conditions.

collagen vascular disease, such as Sjögren's syndrome, rheumatoid arthritis, or systemic lupus erythematosus, or infiltrative disease, such as sarcoidosis. Postradiation treatment of the lacrimal glands, conjunctival scarring from trauma or diseases such as ocular pemphigoid or the Stevens-Johnson syndrome, and vitamin A deficiency also cause severe dry eye, but these conditions will usually be suggested to the doctor from the history or examination. A more common cause of dry eye complaints (although rarely acute ones) is the use of systemic medications such as oral contraceptives, antihistamines, anticholinergics, antidepressants, or beta-blockers. A thorough case history will uncover the use of these.

Blepharitis can give rise to mild to moderate foreign body pain. A history of chronically red, crusty eyes with tearing and burning is typical. The patient will often report recurrences of styes and chalazia. There may also be a concomitant history of rosacea or seborrheic dermatitis. If rosacea is suspected, ask about the presence of chronic skin problems and a history of facial flushing. Ask patients with suspected sebor-

Ask about blepharitis and associated conditions.

rhea if they have skin crusting or scaling. Patients with chronic blepharitis will sometimes present with the acute onset of a red, painful eye due to acute meibomianitis, external or internal hordeolum, corneal ulcer, or corneal infiltrate. A red, tender eye is typical. Photophobia may be present with corneal involvement.

Preseptal cellulitis is marked by pain and redness of the lids. Mild fever may be present. Recent history of internal hordeolum, puncture wound, or sinus infection may be noted. There may be an association with *Staphylococcal* blepharitis. The patient with orbital cellulitis will have pain, red eye, restriction of eye movements, and fever. Visual acuity is often reduced. A history of sinus infection, ocular infection such as dacryocystitis, or trauma is usually associated.

Ask about history of blepharitis, internal hordeolum, puncture wound, or sinus infection if preseptal cellulitis is suspected. Don't forget about orbital cellulitis.

Patients with acute dacryocystitis present with pain, redness, and swelling over the lacrimal sac. Tearing, discharge, and fever may also be present. A history of recurrences is possible.

Patients with conjunctivitis often present emergently because of a red eye but may have minor eye pain or discomfort. Pain is usually not a major pre-

---

Ask about symptoms of discharge, photophobia, and itching in patients with suspected viral or allergic conjunctivitis.

---

senting sign except in severe cases of epidemic keratoconjunctivitis (EKC) and sometimes with significant allergic reactions. Patients with EKC, an adenovirus infection, can present with very red, painful eyes. There is usually a complaint of significant discharge and photophobia, and there may be a history of contact with someone who has a red eye or recent upper respiratory infection. Patients with severe allergic reactions will usually have a history of previous bouts of allergy or a chronic allergy history. Complaints of severe lid and conjunctival swelling are often present. The history in patients with red eyes is discussed in Chapter 14.

Patients with episcleritis or pingueculitis often describe their eyes as feeling uncomfortable rather than painful. They may present after a few days of this discomfort rather than immediately. The patient should be asked about previous episodes of similar problems. Recurrences are associated with an increased likelihood of collagen vascular disease, gout, infection with herpes zoster, herpes simplex, Lyme disease, or syphilis, or other problems such as rosacea or atopic keratoconjunctivitis. A history of arthritis, dermatological problems, or past viral infection should be sought. In most cases, however, patients with episcleritis and pingueculitis have no associated disease history.

Ask about accompanying systemic disease in patients with episcleritis and, particularly, scleritis.

Scleritis is an uncommon condition. Patients with scleritis will present with severe pain and red eye. There is almost always a history of systemic disease such as autoimmune disease, syphilis, tuberculosis, gout, or herpes zoster. Rheumatoid arthritis is particularly common.

Corneal conditions such as abrasion, recurrent erosion, ulcer, and infiltration are frequently associated with significant eye pain because of the abundance of sensory nerve endings in the cornea. Patients should be asked about recent corneal trauma leading to foreign body or abrasion. Corneal erosion can occur weeks after a corneal injury, so an injury history and the type of injury should be sought. Patients with corneal erosion may have relatively severe pain upon awakening and opening their eyes. This history makes the diagnosis of recurrent corneal erosion likely.

Corneal ulcers may be infectious or sterile but will almost always be painful. Patients with bacterial corneal ulcer will present with acute or subacute pain, red eye, and a serous or mucopurulent discharge. A history of contact lens wear is significant due to the increased incidence of infectious corneal ulceration in lens wearers. Corneal ulcers from herpes simplex virus will be painful in those patients who have not had multiple recurrences. These recurrences will damage sensory nerves, leading to loss of sensitivity and diminution of pain. A history of recurrent, unilateral red eye and pain is associated. Sterile ulceration can occur from inflammation, hypoxia, as a response to toxic insult, and from corneal degeneration. In general, infectious ulcers are more painful than sterile ones but this is not always the case and should certainly not be the sole criterion for making this determination.

Corneal infiltrates, accumulations of white blood cells, may appear for any number of reasons but always indicate corneal inflammation. Infiltrates may be peripheral, central, or diffuse. A history of chronic blepharitis, contact lens wear, or viral infection may be associated, but infiltrates can be associated with a variety of causes. Patients with corneal infiltrates may present with a painful, photophobic eye.

Ask about trauma, contact lens wear, history of infection, lid disease, symptoms of pain on awakening, level of pain, and presence of photophobia if corneal disease is suspected.

Nonspecific superficial punctate keratitis will be associated with a scratchy, irritated eye that could cause the patient to present acutely. A history of inflammation, toxic insult, viral infection, or contact lens wear may be associated.

Uveitis is a relatively common cause of eye pain. The acute uveitis patient presents with the sudden onset of a unilateral, painful, red, photophobic eye. This type of presentation is often linked to the HLA-B27 haplotype. HLA-B27 uveitis is associated with idiopathic uveitis, ankylosing spondylitis, and Reiter's syndrome. A history of previous bouts of uveitis, low back pain, or urethritis should be sought. A recurrence of uveitis increases the likelihood of systemic involvement. Other systemic conditions associated with acute, anterior uveitis

Ask about previous episodes and history of other symptoms in patients with suspected acute uveitis.

include inflammatory bowel disease, psoriatic arthritis, Lyme disease, and Behçet's disease. Patients with chronic uveitis and/or bilateral uveitis usually have a more insidious onset of their condition and will present subacutely. There is a much greater chance of finding an association to systemic disease in these patients. Sarcoidosis, syphilis, tuberculosis, and herpes simplex and zoster in adults and juvenile rheumatoid arthritis in children cause chronic, bilateral uveitis.

Patients with the acute onset of elevated IOP from angle-closure glaucoma will present with painful, red eyes, halos around lights, and nausea. Acute angle-closure glaucoma (ACG) is relatively uncommon but is a true urgent ocular condition. Patients with ACG may have a history of intermittent periods of eye pain, blurred vision, or halos around lights from previous bouts of intermittent

Patients with acute ACG will complain of blurred vision, halos around lights, and nausea in addition to pain. Ask them about previous history of pain, blurred vision, or halos.

closure, and will usually have hyperopic refractive error. Patients with elevated IOP associated with ocular inflammation—as in uveitic glaucoma, glaucomatocyclitic crisis, and phacolytic glaucoma—will also present with acute-onset eye pain. A history of previous bouts of pain should be sought. Elevated IOP from noninflammatory open-angle glaucomas will not be associated with eye pain.

Posterior segment disease is usually not associated with pain due to the paucity of sensory nerve innervation in this part of the eye. However, patients with posterior uveitis may have pain. A history of toxoplasmosis, ocular histoplasmosis, sarcoidosis, syphilis, recent surgery, or trauma may be present.

Ask about associated systemic disease, eye surgery, or trauma when posterior uveitis is suspected.

Pain on eye movements associated with an acute onset of unilateral vision loss is typical of optic neuritis. The history, examination, and management of this condition are described in Chapter 17.

Ocular pain associated with diplopia is associated with disease of the orbit, parasellar region, posterior fossa, or migraine. Orbital conditions include orbital pseudotumor, sinusitis, lymphoma, or metastasis. A red, congested, proptotic eye may be seen. Disease of the superior orbital fissure may have a similar presentation. Meningioma, pituitary adenoma, and sinus mucocele is associated with pain from parasellar disease. Posterior communicating artery aneurysm can lead to eye pain in association with ophthalmoplegia as well.

Ask about change in appearance of eyes, headache, and neurological symptoms if pain is associated with diplopia.

Ask about sinus and headache history if referred pain is suspected.

Headache pain and referred pain may also feel like eye pain to the patient and cause him or her to present acutely to the optometrist. Patients with acute sinusitis often complain of pain in and around the eye. A history of previous bouts of sinus problems or a history of allergy or recent viral infection may be present. Migraine or cluster headache sufferers may also have pain referred to their eyes. A headache history is almost always present.

Primary Actions

- Establish the onset, duration, frequency, severity, progression, and quality of the pain.

• Try to determine associated ocular or systemic conditions that may help determine the etiology of the pain.

EXAMINATION

The initial assessment of the patient with eye pain is relatively simple: is the eye red or is it quiet? The red eye implies inflammation while the quiet eye indicates that the etiology may be someplace external to the eye.

> *Initial assessment: is the eye red or quiet?*

If the eye is red, the pattern of the redness should be ascertained. All patients should be first evaluated outside the slit lamp to get a better idea

> *Assess pattern and quality of hyperemia outside the slit lamp.*

of the pattern of the hyperemia. The clinician should note whether the redness is diffuse or localized, its principal location if localized, if it is superficial or deep, and whether there is ciliary injection or flush. The presence of ciliary flush indicates anterior chamber inflammation. As with any red eye, the preauricular lymph nodes should be palpated. Tender, palpable nodes increase the likelihood of an infectious cause for the red eye.

Visual acuity will often be reduced in cases of anterior chamber inflammation, when the central

> *Measure visual acuity.*

cornea is compromised, in cases of acute angle closure glaucoma, when the posterior segment is inflamed, or when there is optic nerve compression. Conditions such as bacterial conjunctivitis, episcleritis, or meibomianitis do not usually affect visual acuity.

Extraocular motilities should be evaluated in all patients with eye pain. Pain on eye movements with acute, unilateral vision loss is typical of optic neuritis. Restricted eye movements in the context of eye pain are associated with congestive orbital conditions such as orbital inflammatory pseudotumor, lymphoma, metastasis, orbital cellulitis, and inflammatory conditions of the superior orbital fissure and anterior cavernous

> *Evaluate EOMs.*

sinus. Thyroid orbitopathy is not painful unless there is corneal exposure. Disease of the parasellar area such as pituitary adenoma, sphenoid sinus mucocele, and meningioma is also part of the differential. Posterior communicating artery aneurysm can cause eye pain and painful ophthalmoplegia as well. Ophthalmoplegic migraine may cause painful diplopia with referred eye pain.

Pupillary examination is useful in these patients as the pupil will often be smaller in the pres-

> *Assess pupillary size and response.*

ence of intraocular inflammation. Additionally, the pupil may be sluggish in cases of orbital disease due to optic nerve compression. The pupil will be non-reactive and middilated in patients with acute angle-closure glaucoma.

In the majority of cases, the diagnosis will be based on the findings at the slit lamp. The differential will follow different paths depending on whether the patient has a red eye or the eye is quiet.

Red Eye

The presence or absence of hyperemia and its pattern if present should be assessed before the patient is placed behind the slit lamp. The slit lamp examination should then be used to determine its cause.

Red eye with mild to moderate pain is typical of lid and conjunctival disease. Dry eye syndrome, blepharitis, blepharoconjunctivitis, conjunctivitis, pingueculitis, and episcleritis are likely. Nonspecific superficial punctate keratitis (SPK) should also be considered. Moderate to severe pain is more typical of corneal disease, anterior uveitis, scleritis, and angle-closure glaucoma.

Mild-to-Moderate Pain

Evaluation for dry eye should be done with standard tests such as observation of the lacrimal lake, tear breakup time, Schirmer testing, and staining of the conjunctiva and cornea with fluorescein, rose Ben-

Evaluate the tear film.

gal, or lissamine green dyes. If dry eye is the cause of the patient's pain, corneal staining will be present.

The lids should be examined for the presence of blepharitis. Significant blepharitis is uncomfortable and can lead to more painful eye conditions such as meibomianitis, external and internal hordeola,

Assess lids for blepharitis and complications of blepharitis.

and *Staphylococcal* blepharokeratoconjunctivitis. Tender, clogged meibomian gland orifices are signs of meibomianitis. Hordeola will present as an area of localized lid redness and elevation that is tender to the touch. Internal hordeola are much more uncomfortable; patients will tend to jump back when the hordeola is palpated. *Staphylococcal* blepharokeratoconjunctivitis can result in tender and ulcerated lids, corneal punctate staining, marginal corneal infiltrates, or corneal ulceration (Figure 15–1).

Assess lids, presence of proptosis, and EOMs in patients with preseptal cellulitis.

Patients with preseptal cellulitis will have a red, tender eyelid that is warm to the touch. Conjunctival chemosis will often be present. Proptosis, pain on eye movements, and restriction of eye

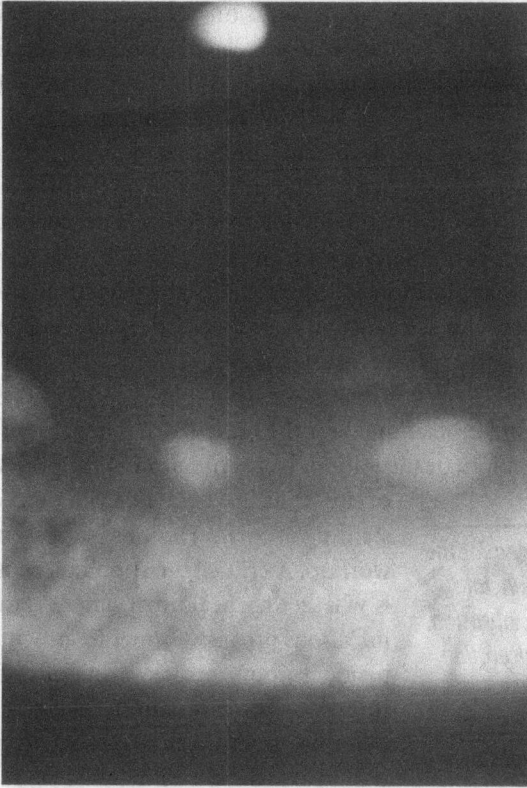

Figure 15–1. Marginal corneal infiltrates in a patient with staphylococcal blepharitis.

movements will not be present as they will be in orbital cellulitis. Preseptal cellulitis in young children is associated with a great deal of upper and lower eyelid edema and a purple coloration of the lid.

Dacryocystitis will cause pain, redness, and swelling in the region of the medial canthus. Pressure over the lacrimal sac will cause a purulent discharge to be expressed from the puncta.

> Try to express discharge from the puncta in suspected dacryocystitis.

Sectoral hyperemia is the hallmark finding of episcleritis, though episcleritis can also appear as diffuse redness. Episcleritis can usually be differentiated from conjunctivitis by lack of mucopurulent discharge and limitation of the hyperemia to the bulbar area. Engorgement will be noted in the larger episcleral vessels that run radially beneath the conjunctiva. The clinician should also look for nodules, which are localized accumulations of inflammatory material. The nodules will appear as whitish, slightly

Determine if the episcleral or scleral vessels are engorged and if nodules are present.

mobile elevations within the area of inflammation. Nodular episcleritis increases the likelihood that the episcleritis will be associated with an underlying systemic disease, although in most cases both simple and nodular episcleritis are not associated with systemic illness. Episcleritis can be differentiated from scleritis because the injection in scleritis is deeper and is blue or violaceous in color, particularly with room illumination. The scleral vessels will not blanch upon application of topical 2.5% phenylephrine. As stated previously, the patient with scleritis will have severe, deep, boring pain.

Moderate-to-Severe Pain

The cornea should be examined for the presence of punctate keratitis, erosion, abrasion, infiltration, or ulceration. Determination of the presence or absence of fluorescein, rose Bengal, or lissamine green staining of corneal lesions is an essential part of the workup. A critical question that must be answered is whether corneal involvement is due to an active infectious process. Proper treatment is entirely dependent upon the answering of this question. An infectious process is more likely with greater hyperemia, anterior chamber reaction, and infiltration in association with higher degrees of pain, discharge, and history of contact lens wear. If the clinician cannot answer the question of whether the condition is infectious or not with certainty, the patient must be treated as if he or she has an infection.

Examine the cornea for the presence of punctate keratitis, erosion, abrasion, infiltration, or ulceration.

Determine corneal staining patterns.

Determine if there is a corneal infection.

Discovery of corneal dendrites in one eye (dendritic keratitis) is pathognomonic for herpes simplex virus (HSV) infection (see Figure 14–3). HSV infection, however, may also present as unilateral SPK or widespread (ameboid, geographic) ulceration as well. The epithelial lesions of suspected HSV keratitis need to be carefully examined without and with vital dyes. The base of true dendrites will stain profusely with fluorescein (they are ulcers) while rose Bengal will outline the edges of the ulcer. True terminal end bulbs will be present. Stromal inflammation may appear alone or together with epithelial keratitis. This inflammation may appear as stromal haze that may be associated with endothelial folds, anterior chamber cells and flare, and elevated IOP. Stromal keratitis is an immune response to viral antigen.

Patients with corneal infiltrative reactions may present with the acute onset of pain, redness, and photophobia. Corneal infiltrates may be seen as part of any process in which the immune system has been activated in response to corneal insult. Infiltrates may occur due to hypoxia, in response to toxic insult, after viral infection in epidemic keratoconjunctivitis, as part of a hypersensitivity reaction, or as part of the response to an infectious agent. Infiltrate associated with infectious keratitis is dense and underlies the area of ulceration, and is associated with anterior chamber reaction and with greater amounts of hyperemia. Sterile infiltrates tend to cause less symptomatology, may be multiple, and occur in association with an intact or nearly intact epithelium. Infiltrates associated with *Staphylococcus* hypersensitivity tend to be peripheral (marginal) and multiple in patients with blepharitis (Figure 15–1).

IOP should be measured in all patients with ocular pain. The acute onset of a red, painful eye in association with high intraocular pressure and a narrow anterior chamber angle is most likely acute angle-closure glaucoma. The cornea may be edematous ("steamy") making it difficult to examine the anterior chamber and angle. The addition of a topical hyperosmolar

> *Measure IOP and perform gonioscopy if the IOP is elevated.*

agent such as glycerin, 0.5% solution, can be instilled to reduce corneal edema and make examination easier. Gonioscopy must be performed to determine if the angle is truly closed (Figure 15–2). Compression gonioscopy can determine if the angle is synechially closed and to help break the attack. The contralateral angle should also be examined; patients with primary angle-closure glaucoma will have narrow angles in both eyes whereas a secondary cause is indicated in the patient with an open angle opposite the closed one. Other causes of acute angle-closure glaucoma include neovascular glaucoma and

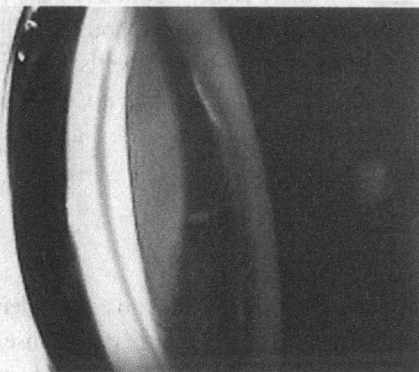

Figure 15–2. Gonioscopic appearance of closed angle in acute ACG.

those associated with mechanical closure of the angle such as phacomorphic glaucoma, choroidal detachment, or posterior segment tumor. Acute angle-closure glaucoma is a true ocular urgency and the optometrist should be well versed in its diagnosis and treatment.

Examine anterior chamber for cells, flare, hyphema, and hypopyon.

A painful eye with ciliary flush is indicative of anterior chamber inflammation. The degree of cells and flare should be graded on a scale of trace to 4+. The presence of pigment or blood in the anterior chamber should also be noted. Keratic precipitates (KPs) should be inspected to differentiate nongranulomatous from granulomatous uveitis. In general, fine KPs are seen as part of nongranulomatous uveitis whereas large, "mutton-fat" KPs are seen with granulomatous. In granulomatous uveitis, the iris may have nodules on the pupillary border (Koeppe) or on the anterior iris surface (Busacca).

Examine the lens for cataract and for its relationship to anterior segment structures.

It is important that the posterior part of the eye be examined in patients with painful, red eyes as well. The presence of significant cataract can have a major impact on the state of the anterior chamber. Patients with narrow angles, high IOP, and mature cataracts likely have a phacomorphic component to their angle closure. Removal of the lens will need to be a part of the care of this type of patient. Patients with anterior chamber cells and flare and a mature or hypermature cataract may have phacolytic uveitis or, if the IOP is elevated, phacolytic glaucoma. This occurs due to leakage of lens proteins and subsequent inflammatory reaction.

Examine posterior pole if the diagnosis is in doubt.

If the clinician is sure of the diagnosis, dilated examination of the vitreous and retina may not have to be performed at the initial visit. However, if there is any doubt as to the cause of the painful, red eye the pupils should be dilated and the posterior segment evaluated for signs of posterior uveitis. Signs include vitritis, retinal or choroidal infiltration, vascular sheathing, posterior segment edema, disc swelling, and retinal hemorrhages and exudates. Signs of anterior segment inflammation may appear as well.

Quiet Eye

The white, painful eye can be a greater diagnostic challenge because the less dramatic presentation may not directly identify the cause of the problem.

Intraepithelial corneal infiltrates in the presence of a white eye are diagnostic of Thygeson's superficial punctate keratopathy. This condition, which tends to exacerbate and remit over many years, is marked by periodic acute flare-ups. During the period of acute exacerbation, the eye

Examine cornea in patients with white, painful eyes.

may not be totally white despite classical teaching. Fluorescein staining will highlight the location of these lesions. During quiescent periods, the infiltrates may disappear, or may be present but not affect the superficial epithelium. Negative staining may then occur at the site of the lesions.

The patient presenting with pain on eye movements and acute loss of visual acuity must be suspected of having optic neuritis. The examination of these patients is covered in Chapter 17.

Painful Ophthalmoplegia

Persons with painful ophthalmoplegia may present with quiet or red eyes, significant pain, and constant diplopia or diplopia in particular fields of gaze (Figure 15–3). After ascertaining which muscles are involved, the clinician should attempt to determine whether the ophthalmoplegia is due to orbital dis-

In painful ophthalmoplegia, determine if the orbit is involved.

ease. The cardinal signs of orbital disease include pain, proptosis, resistance to retropulsion, diplopia, and reduced vision. Exophthalmometry measurements should be recorded and direct pressure should be applied through closed lids to determine if the eye can be retropulsed. If orbital disease is suspected, MRI of the orbit is indicated. Potential causes of painful, orbital disease include inflammatory pseudotumor, orbital cellulitis, tumor metastasis, orbital lymphoma, and orbital vasculitis. Patients with disease of the superior orbital fissure or anterior cavernous sinus will have multiple cranial nerve palsies in addition to the eye pain. Parasellar disease and posterior fossa disease will have associated visual field defects.

Primary Actions—Examination of the Patient with Eye Pain

- Determine if the eye is red or quiet.
- Tailor the examination based upon the answer to the first primary action.
- Determine if the eye is infected.
- Determine if any urgent conditions are present.

A

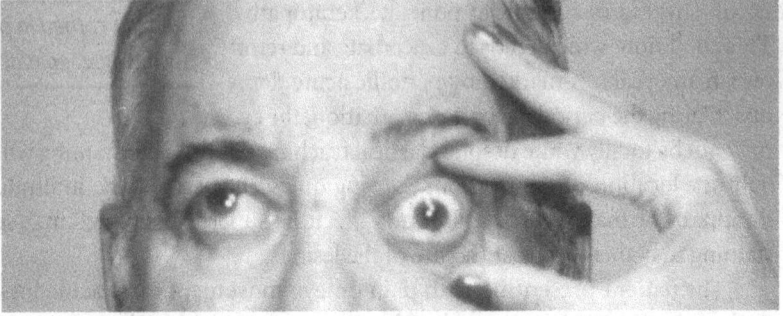

B

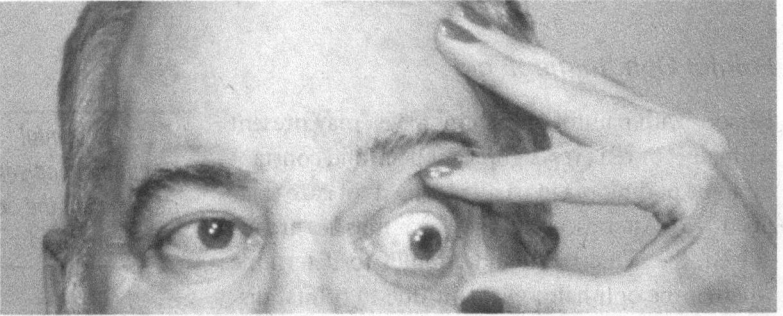

Figure 15–3. (A and B). Restricted eye movements in a patient with painful ophthalmoplegia due to the Tolosa-Hunt syndrome.

MANAGEMENT

In patients with acute exacerbation of dry eye, the eye condition must be treated with copious amounts of unpreserved or minimally preserved artificial tears. If there is significant corneal staining, antibiotic drops or mild ointments can be added. A trial of punctal occlusion with collagen or silicone punctal plugs is indicated. In patients with underlying inflammatory disease, cyclosporine, 0.05% emulsion (Restasis) bid, may prove useful. This product recently received FDA approval. As exacerbation of the dry eye may be a marker for increased activity of the systemic disease, consultation with the patient's physician is indicated in these cases.

Aggressively treat dry eye and comanage associated systemic disease.

The patient presenting with outright pain from lid disease and associated pathology will require more than lid scrubs to alleviate the problem. Warm compresses with lid massage will be needed to treat acute meibomianitis to allow drainage from the meibomian gland orifices, but this will need to be supplemented with topical antibiotic drops and bedtime ointment to prevent secondary conjunctivitis. Combination antibiotic-steroid drops or ointment will be needed if the lids are markedly inflamed. A recommended regimen would be warm

> *Treat acutely symptomatic lid disease with warm compresses and lid massage, broad-spectrum antibiotics, or antibiotic-steroid combinations.*

compresses with lid massage for 15 minutes, three or four times per day, broad-spectrum antibiotic drops qid, and erythromycin or bacitracin ointment at bedtime. Antibiotic-steroid combination therapy may be substituted for either the antibiotic drops or ointment if the practitioner chooses. Combinations of low-dose prednisolone-sulfacetamide and tobramycin-dexamethasone used in drop form qid and bedtime ointment have been used successfully. Long-term therapy includes lid hygiene, supplemental artificial tears, and, in recalcitrant cases or those associated with underlying rosacea, an oral tetracycline such as doxycycline used over the course of months. For example, 100 mg doxycycline can be used bid for two to three months and tapered to once a day for another two to three months. Obviously, this is just a guideline that can be adjusted depending on clinical appearance.

Mild-to-moderate preseptal cellulitis in persons older than age five should be treated with antibiotics with activity against the organisms that are most likely to cause the infection, *Staphylococcus aureus* or streptococci. First-generations cephalosporins, amoxicillin/clavulanate, erythromycin, and trimethoprim/sulfamethoxazole are all suitable. Moderate-to-severe preseptal cellulitis, or preseptal cellulitis in children younger than age five, when *Hemophilus* infection is suspected, or when the patient is not improving, should be treated with intravenous antibiotics in the hospital. Ceftriaxone and vancomycin is the treatment of choice.

Marginal corneal infiltrates from *Staphylococcus* require lid treatment plus treatment of the corneal lesions. These infiltrates respond readily to topical steroids. Combination antibiotic-steroid treatment is usually the simplest and most convenient for the patient. A reasonable approach is lid hygiene plus combination steroid-antibiotic drop therapy qid or more often depending on the symptoms and amount of inflammation. If there is significant meibomian gland

> *Treat marginal corneal infiltrates with antibiotic-steroid combination.*

stasis this needs to be treated with warm compresses and digital lid massage.

Treatment of corneal pathology needs to be focused on the underlying cause. The clinician should always remember the risk of significant vision loss from corneal infection or inflammation.

Superficial punctate keratitis (SPK) is a nonspecific finding and treatment should be aimed at the underlying etiology. Patients with SPK should be treated with unpreserved or minimally preserved artificial tears in addition to specific treatment for the underlying condition if it is known. There are times when the SPK is a stand-alone finding; in these cases use of tears and careful monitoring for the appearance of other findings may be all that is needed. Significant SPK or SPK in a contact lens wearer may require prophylactic treatment with a broad-spectrum antibiotic if the practitioner is concerned about bacterial infection; qid treatment is usually sufficient in these cases.

Treat SPK with unpreserved or minimally preserved artificial tears or broad-spectrum antibiotics.

Patients with corneal ulceration from suspected infectious causes need to be treated aggressively (Table 15–2). The clinician must decide if the patient with bacterial keratitis can be treated empirically with topical drops, whether fortified antibiotics are needed, and whether the lesion should be cultured. Although culture with sensitivity will identify the causative organism and antibiotic susceptibility, most offices do not have the means to do this. If the optometrist feels that the ulcer puts the patient at major risk for vision loss, the patient should be sent to a cornea specialist for care that should include culture and sensitivity and treatment with fortified antibiotics. If the clinician feels that he wishes to treat the patient himself, aggressive treatment with fluoroquinolone drops should be started immediately. A loading dose of one drop every 15 minutes for the first two hours followed by q1h dosing is indicated although the manufacturer's instructions and other treatment protocols may differ slightly.

Treat bacterial keratitis with topical fluoroquinolones or fortified antibiotics and cycloplegics. Follow the next day.

At this time, ciprofloxacin and ofloxacin are the only fluoroquinolone drops approved for treatment of bacterial keratitis; it is expected that fourth-generation fluoroquinolones (moxifloxacin and gatifloxacin) will supplant treatment with current fluoroquinolones when they are approved. Some practitioners recommend around-the-clock treatment with fluoroquinolones for at least the first day to maintain therapeutic concentrations. An alternative treatment is the use of bedtime ointment. Although ciprofloxacin ointment is available, it is our recommendation that a different antibiotic be used to increase the chance of successful treatment in cases of fluoroquinolone resistance. Polymyxin B–bacitracin ointment is a broad-spectrum antibiotic with good coverage against most bacteria associated with bacterial keratitis and little bacterial resistance. Use of an ointment allows the patient to sleep, which will improve the immune response to the infection. Cycloplegic drops, such as 5% homatropine, 1% cyclopento-

Table 15–2   Treatment of Bacterial Keratitis

Fluoroquinolone treatment—topical ciprofloxacin or ofloxacin
  Loading dose—one drop q 15 minutes × 2 hours or other
    One drop q1h while awake
  Polysporin ointment at bedtime
  Reassess the next day
  Maintain q1h–q2h for next several days depending on severity and response to
    treatment
  Introduce topical steroid drops when improvement seen and re-epithelialization is
    taking place
Fortified antibiotic treatment
  Fortified tobramycin or gentamycin, 15 mg /mL every hour, alternated with
  Fortified cefazolin, 50 mg/mL, or fortified vancomycin, 25 mg/mL every hour

late, or 0.25% scopolamine, should be used bid or tid to improve comfort. Pain relief in the form of acetaminophen may also be recommended.

Patients with bacterial keratitis treated in-office must be seen the next day. It would not be surprising to see little if any improvement in the clinical appearance of the lesion, but the patient may report some improvement in symptoms. No change in treatment is recommended at this point. On the second day the clinical appearance of the lesion and the patient discomfort should be improved. The clinician may wish to decrease drop frequency to q2h depending on the initial results to treatment, location of the lesion, size of the lesion, and amount of infiltrate. The patient needs to be followed carefully with reduction of frequency of medications and longer intervals between visits as the patient shows improvement.

The use of topical steroids in bacterial keratitis must also be considered here. Traditional thinking says that steroids should not be introduced until the cornea has completely re-epithelialized. However, if there is significant underlying infiltrate, the epithelium may never completely heal and persistent fluorescein staining defects will be present. Topical corticosteroid will break up the infiltrate and prevent scarring and allow the epithelium to recover. Introduction of topical steroids should be considered when the infection appears to be under control and signs of re-epithelialization are evident. Steroids can be introduced at q4h and must always be used concurrently with topical antibiotic. A switch to a topical antibiotic-steroid drop and ointment is appropriate after the infection is under control.

> *Consider topical steroids as part of the treatment of infectious bacterial keratitis.*

Herpes simplex epithelial keratitis also needs to be treated promptly upon diagnosis. Although herpetic dendrites will heal without treatment, appropriate antiviral therapy is indicated to speed resolution and reduce corneal damage from infection and the immune response to the infection. Standard treatment of HSV epithelial keratitis is trifluridine 1% drops q2h up to nine times per day for no longer than 21 days. On average, this treatment will completely clear up dendrites in about six days. Supplemental cycloplegia will increase patient comfort. Patients should be followed in 24 to 48 hours for treatment response. The optometrist should remember that trifluridine is toxic to the cornea and nonherpetic SPK may develop. This should not be considered treatment failure. Alternative treatments for HSV epithelial keratitis include vidarabine ointment five times per day and acyclovir ointment three times per day. The latter treatment is not approved for this use in the United States but is in many other countries. Debridement was the treatment of choice before the advent of topical antiviral agents and is still recommended by many practitioners alone or in combination with antiviral ointment therapy and patching. Debridement removes infected epithelial cells and dead, sloughed-off tissue, allowing for control of infection and improved corneal healing. Loose epithelium can be wiped away with a cotton-tipped applicator after topical anesthesia. We recommend debridement in those cases in which there is a great deal of heaped-up, dead epithelium that will prove to be an obstacle to healing.

Treat HSV epithelial keratitis with topical antiviral agent (and debridement).

Some patients with HSV will have stromal keratitis, which may follow epithelial keratitis, occur concurrently with it, or occur alone. In most cases, stromal keratitis will occur in patients who have had previous bouts of HSV disease, but it can occur as an initial disease presentation. The clinician must recognize stromal keratitis as a forerunner of vision loss in the patient with HSV disease, as it can lead to scarring, chronic inflammation, and IOP elevation, and is associated with increased risk of recurrence. Stromal keratitis is an inflammatory response to viral antigen and needs to be treated with topical anti-inflammatory treatment. Usual treatment is topical prednisolone acetate drops whose frequency of administration depends on the magnitude of the inflammation. As topical steroids will increase or activate viral replication, topical or oral antiviral agents need to be utilized as well. Usual administration is trifluridine drops qid or oral acyclovir 200–400 mg five times a day. The antiviral agents can be tapered in step with the steroid taper. A slow taper is recommended, particularly in patients who have had previous recurrences of stromal disease.

Treat stromal keratitis with topical steroids and antiviral cover.

Prevention of recurrence of HSV keratitis will prevent vision loss and research in recent years has aimed to find ways to prevent these recurrences. The Herpes Eye Disease Study (HEDS) showed that 400 mg bid oral acyclovir used for one year in patients with previously treated HSV eye disease reduces the rate of recurrence of all cases of HSV disease by 38% and the risk of stromal keratitis by 50% in patients at risk for stromal keratitis. We recommend long-term oral acyclovir 400 mg bid in those patients at risk for recurrence and vision loss: patients with previous recurrences and patients with previous bouts of stromal keratitis.

> *Use 400 mg oral acyclovir bid for one year to reduce the risk of HSV recurrence in patients at greatest risk of recurrence.*

HEDS has not answered the question of how long the protective effect of one year of acyclovir lasts: whether it is for just one year or much longer. These answers are forthcoming. We also do not know whether long-term use of the newer oral antivirals famciclovir or valacyclovir is equally efficacious as acyclovir.

Treatment of episcleritis is usually based upon the level of patient symptomatology. Patients with minimal symptoms may be treated with artificial tears and vasoconstrictors. More symptomatic patients usually require topical nonsteroidal anti-inflammatories or topical steroids. We have had very good results using topical loteprednol, 0.2%, tid-qid for 10 to 14 days in symptomatic patients. Loteprednol, 0.2%, is approved for seasonal allergic conjunctivitis but has proven useful off-label for surface inflammatory disease. Topical di-

> *Treat episcleritis based on the degree of patient symptoms. Mild topical steroid is a very effective treatment.*

clofenac, ketorolac, loteprednol, 0.5%, rimexolone, and fluorometholone are also effective. If the patient is not allergic and can tolerate oral ibuprofen, this can be recommended at labeled dosages. Systemic workup of patients with episcleritis is necessary only in recurrent cases or in those not responsive to treatment. Workup focuses on inflammatory disease such as gout and rheumatoid arthritis, and previous history of herpes zoster.

The primary care optometrist should not undertake the management of patients with scleritis alone. Comanagement or outright referral to secondary/tertiary providers such as rheumatologists, cornea specialists, or providers skilled in the management of ocular inflammatory disease is highly recommended. The

> *Diagnose and refer patients with scleritis.*

primary care provider's job is to diagnose scleritis and recognize its relationship to significant vision loss and systemic disease.

Acute angle-closure glaucoma must be treated urgently (Table 15–3). Im-

Table 15-3 Treatment of Acute Angle-Closure Glaucoma

Topical aqueous suppressants if not contraindicated—repeat hourly if IOP does not decrease

   Timolol, 0.5%, one dose

   Iopidine, 0.5%, one dose

   Dorzolamide, 2%, one dose

Oral CAI

   Two 250-mg acetazolamide tablets

Topical pilocarpine, 1% or 2%, q15min for 1 hour, then every hour (if phakic pupillary block or angle crowding)

Topical prednisolone acetate, 1%, q15min for 1 hour, then every hour

If IOP reduction truly urgent (vision loss is imminent):

Oral glycerin, 50% solution, at a dose of 2–3 mg/kg or oral isosorbide in dose of 1–2 g/kg in diabetics

IV mannitol, 20%, at a dose of 1–2 g/kg

Definitive treatment: laser PI when IOP is controlled, angle is open, and inflammation is controlled

---

> *Treat acute ACG with topical aqueous suppressors, pilocarpine, steroids, and oral CAIs. The ultimate treatment is LPI.*

mediate therapy aims to rapidly lower IOP to preserve vision. Aqueous suppressants such as topical beta-blockers, alpha-agonists, and carbonic anhydrase inhibitors, provided there are no contraindications to their use, can be used to lower IOP. Two 250-mg oral acetazolamide tablets (not slower-acting sequels) can be used as well if the IOP is very high. In the case of phakic pupillary block or angle crowding, topical pilocarpine, 1% or 2%, is instilled often over the first two hours. Topical steroids, such as prednisolone acetate, 1%, is instilled every 15 minutes for one hour and then hourly to reduce inflammation. Intermittent pressure on the eye with a gonioscopy lens also may cause reversal. Pupillary block should then be eliminated as soon as possible. The definitive treatment of pupillary block is via laser peripheral iridotomy, which should be performed as soon as the IOP has been lowered to a satisfactory level, usually below that of the contralateral eye, the angle is open gonioscopically, and the eye is no longer inflamed. The contralateral eye should be treated as well, as there is a high risk of developing acute ACG in this eye.

Intermittent angle-closure glaucoma can be treated with laser peripheral iridotomy on a less urgent basis. IOP should be lowered by medical means before the procedure if it is above 30 mmHg. These patients will usually require chronic IOP-lowering agents, similar to patients with primary open-angle glaucoma (POAG), due to outflow problems associated with the long-term meshwork obstruction.

Acute, unilateral, anterior uveitis is treated with topical steroid drops and cycloplegia. Inflammation should be treated aggressively with frequent steroid drops with rapid taper as the inflammation is controlled. Prednisolone acetate q1h–2h is recommended as a starting point in most cases with bid or tid cycloplegia with cyclopentolate, homatropine, or scopolamine. Some practitioners advocate the use of steroids such as rimexolone or loteprednol, which have a lower risk of causing an IOP elevation when compared with prednisolone acetate but still give adequate anti-inflammatory activity. Any IOP elevation secondary to the inflammation should be treated with topical aqueous suppressants if the practitioner feels the disc is at risk for damage at that level of IOP.

> *Treat acute anterior uveitis with aggressive topical steroid treatment and cycloplegia.*

> *If indicated, treat elevated IOP with aqueous suppressants.*

Most cases of acute, unilateral, anterior uveitis are idiopathic in nature and do not require systemic evaluation. Recurrent cases, those unresponsive to treatment, and bilateral cases are more often associated with systemic disease and deserve systemic workup.

The systemic evaluation of acute, unilateral, anterior uveitis should concentrate on those conditions most associated with this type of presentation: the HLA-B27 uveitidies. Reiter's syndrome is evaluated by conjunctival and urethral cultures for *Chlamydia* and joint X-ray if arthritis is present. Radiographs of the sacroiliac spine should be ordered in patients with suspected ankylosing spondylitis. Workup for other etiologies can be performed if signs and symptoms indicate (Table 15–4).

> *Systemic work-up is indicated for recurrent, unresponsive, and bilateral cases of anterior uveitis.*

The mature cataract can lead to elevated IOP because its size causes shallowing of the anterior chamber–phacomorphic glaucoma. The ultimate treatment is removal of the cataract; however, medical treatment of elevated IOP may be required on a short-term basis. Laser peripheral iridotomy may be performed prior to cataract removal to eliminate pupillary block or as a substitute for cataract surgery in cases in which the visual acuity is relatively good or when the patient does not wish cataract surgery.

> *Refer for cataract surgery in most cases of lens-induced narrow-angle glaucoma.*

Phacolytic uveitis and glaucoma is treated acutely by reducing inflammation with topical steroid drops and reducing IOP with aqueous suppressants.

Table 15–4   Systemic Workup of Patients with Acute, Anterior Uveitis

CBC
ESR
ACE
ANA
RPR or VDRL
FTA-ABS
PPD
Chest X-ray
Lyme titer
HLA-B27
Sacroiliac spine radiograph (if ankylosing spondylitis suspected)
Conjunctival and urethral cultures (if Reiter's syndrome suspected)

Note: order those tests only for conditions in which clinical suspicion exists.

The lens needs to be removed as soon as inflammation and IOP are under adequate control.

Management of posterior segment uveitis is aimed at uncovering the underlying cause of the inflammation. Treatment is specific for each condition.

Quiet Eye

Topical steroid drops are the usual treatment for acute exacerbations of Thygeson's superficial keratopathy. Fluorometholone acetate, 1%, qid for 1 to 2 weeks with slow taper has been used successfully to improve patient comfort and reduce inflammation. The practitioner should monitor IOP during the periods of steroid use even though this steroid causes IOP elevation less frequently than prednisolone or dexamethasone. Topical cyclosporine drops, 1% or 2%, have been used successfully after topical steroid failure because of their immunomodulatory and anti-inflammatory properties. These drops have to be specially formulated by a pharmacy. Recently 0.05% cyclosporine (Restasis) has been approved for the treatment of dry eye secondary to inflammation; it is unknown how this much lower concentration will work in the treatment of Thygeson's.

Treat Thygeson's superficial keratopathy with topical steroids.

The management of acute optic neuritis is discussed in Chapter 17.

As painful ophthalmoplegia is associated with a number of ominous conditions, treatment is often comanaged with other medical practitioners. MRI of the orbit should be ordered by the optometrist or through the patient's primary medical provider. If the results indicate lymphoma or metastatic disease, the patient will need to be seen by an oncol-

> *Comanage patients with painful ophthalmoplegia.*

ogist. Orbital pseudotumor is treated with high-dose oral steroids. Rapid response to the steroid is considered diagnostic for orbital pseudotumor but the practitioner must remember that lymphoma may also respond to steroids. The management of the patient with painful ophthalmoplegia is challenging and will often require the expertise of a secondary or tertiary care provider.

Primary Actions—Management of the Patient with Eye Pain

- Manage the specific cause of the eye pain.
- Treat infectious keratitis aggressively.
- Treat inflammation aggressively.
- Consider systemic evaluation in patients with recurrent, unresponsive, or bilateral anterior uveitis.
- Comanage patients with systemic disease with the patient's primary care provider or a secondary or tertiary care specialist.

Chapter 16

Transient Vision Loss

"Doctor, I lost the vision in my eye for a few minutes but it came back. Does this mean anything?"

SCOPE OF THE PROBLEM

Transient vision loss can be a harbinger of significant cardiovascular or cerebrovascular disease. Patients with temporary loss of vision will often present to the optometrist for evaluation. Accurate assessment is needed to determine which of these patients require further medical evaluation and which can be reassured and followed (Table 16–1).

HISTORY

Temporary loss of vision in one or both eyes can be an extremely harrowing experience for some patients, causing them to present to the office immediately. Others may ignore this problem even after it occurs many times, presenting only after multiple events or even mentioning it in passing in a routine examination. Because of the potential significance of this symptom, the clinician must fully investigate it and attempt to determine its cause. Management will be guided by etiology.

The history in patients with transient vision loss should establish the temporal profile of the event. Laterality of the vision loss and whether other body systems were affected at the time of the temporary blindness should also be investigated. Clear answers to these questions will often enable the clinician to determine the etiology and significance of the problem.

Establish the temporal profile and laterality of the vision loss.

Table 16–1   Causes of Transient Vision Loss

Migraine and vasospasm
   Migraine with aura
   Migraine aura without headache
   Retinociliary migraine
Disease of extracranial vessels
   Emboli released from the carotid system
   Stenosis/occlusion of the carotid system
   Emboli from the vertebrobasilar system
   Stenosis/occlusion of the vertebrobasilar system
Cardiac disease
   Atrial fibrillation
   Valvular disease
      Rheumatic heart disease
      Mitral valve disease
      Prosthetic valves
      Endocarditis
      Calcific aortic stenosis
   Myocardial infarct
   Atrial myxoma
   Cardiomyopathy
   Cardiac insufficiency
Hyperviscosity syndromes
Hypercoagulable states
Local ocular causes
   Optic disc edema
   Optic disc anomalies
   Intermittent angle-closure glaucoma
   Vitreous debris
   Tear film abnormalities
   Blepharospasm
   Orbital mass

Vision loss lasting 15 minutes or more, characterized by a small scotoma that enlarges over time, is typical of migraine. Fortification spectra around the scotoma (scintillating scotoma) or distortions within the area of vision loss are common. There may be associated focal neurological deficits such as sensory or motor losses or cognitive impairment.

> *Ask about fortification spectra, focal neurological deficits, or associated neurological symptoms.*

The clinician should always remember that

Table 16–2 International Headache Society Headache Classification

---

Primary or nonorganic headache
  Migraine
  Tension-type headache
  Cluster headache
  Miscellaneous
Secondary or organic
  Trauma
  Vascular disorders
  Nonvascular intracranial disorders
  Intracranial inflammation
  Substance abuse and withdrawal
  Noncephalic infection
  Metabolic disorders
  Disorders of facial and cranial structures
  Cranial neuralgias, nerve trunk pain, and deafferentation pain
  Nonclassifiable
Classification of migraine
  Migraine with aura ("classic migraine")
  Migraine without aura ("common migraine")
  Migraine aura without headache ("acephalgic migraine")
  Retinociliary migraine ("ocular migraine")
  Ophthalmoplegic migraine
  Basilar migraine
  Chronic daily headache
  Lower-half headache
  Migraine with prolonged aura
  Familial hemiplegic migraine

Headache Classification Committee of the International Headache Society. Classification and diagnostic criteria for headache disorders, cranial neuralgias, and facial pain. *Cephalalgia* 1988; 8(suppl 7):1.

headache is not a necessary component of migraine. Migraine is a symptom complex and may include the homonymous field loss characteristic of migraine headache with aura (classic migraine) and migraine aura without headache (acephalgic migraine), or unilateral vision loss seen with cilioretinal migraine (see the International Headache Society classification of headache for a complete description of these terms—Table 16–2).

Most forms of migraine are brain-related phenomena; therefore, it is expected that the vision loss characteristic of migraine be bilateral, homonymous loss. However, many patients often have difficulty in determining whether vision loss is in a homonymous hemifield or in one eye, so laterality is not as important an indicator as the temporal profile of the event. Regardless of laterality, vision loss of 15 minutes or more with escalating symptoms is highly suggestive of migraine.

Care must be taken in caring for older patients with new-onset migraine, as migraine typically begins early in life (often puberty) and diminishes over time. However, it is not unheard of for an older patient to develop migraine. The clinician must decide if he or she is comfortable in making the diagnosis of new-onset migraine in an older patient. If the clinician has any doubt, further evaluation is warranted.

Transient vision loss of greater than 15 minutes without escalation of symptoms, with or without headache, may be migraine but also could be indicative of cerebral lesions such as arteriovenous malformations or meningiomas. Vision loss associated with structural lesions may begin transiently, but will usually become permanent over time.

Ask about bilateral symptoms consistent with vertebrobasilar insufficiency.

Bilateral vision loss lasting a few minutes may be due to ischemia in the vertebrobasilar (posterior) circulation. As blood to the posterior part of the brain comes from the paired vertebral arteries, transient vision loss caused by vertebrobasilar insufficiency is usually bilateral. These patients may have other neurological and ocular signs and symptoms consistent with ischemia of the posterior circulation to the brain and should be questioned about sensory or motor loss, nausea, vomiting, dysarthria, dysphagia, and diplopia (Table 16–3).

Unilateral vision loss lasting from two to 15 minutes but typically three to five minutes is called amaurosis fugax, or fleeting blindness. Besides its unilateral nature and temporal profile, amaurosis fugax is marked by sectoral or altitudinal vision loss that mimics the vascular pattern of the retina, and a return to its previous status as quickly as it came. The vision loss may be complete or may be described as a blurring, fogging, or graying.

Specifically ask about the symptoms that are stereotypical for amaurosis fugax.

Amaurosis fugax is caused by emboli lodging in the retinal vessels for a short period of time and then moving downstream. Usually, these emboli are released from the ipsilateral carotid artery. Amaurosis fugax is the most common symptom of carotid artery disease and is virtually pathognomonic for this condition if accurately diagnosed. It is highly associated with complex, acoustically heterogeneous carotid plaques, which are those most likely to release emboli.

Ask patient with amaurosis fugax about global neurological symptoms.

Amaurosis fugax must be recognized as an oc-

Table 16-3 Transient Ischemic Attacks (TIAs)

Carotid territory
  Ipsilateral vision loss
  Contralateral hemiparesis
  Contralateral hemisensory loss
  Aphasia (if dominant hemisphere)
  Sensory neglect (if nondominant hemisphere)
  Homonymous hemianopia
Vertebrobasilar territory
  Bilateral vision loss
  Quadraparesis
  Bilateral sensory and motor deficits
  Perioral numbness
  Falls without loss of consciousness (drop attacks)
  Diplopia
  Vertigo
  Syncope
  Dysarthria
  Nausea
  Dysphagia

ular transient ischemic attack (TIA). The patient should be questioned about the presence of contralateral numbness or weakness and difficulty in speech indicative of widespread cerebral ischemia (Table 16-3).

Sudden, unilateral transient vision loss may also be caused by emboli released from the heart as well as the carotid, although cardiac emboli are more often associated with the permanent vision loss seen with retinal artery occlusion. Potential

> *Ask about symptoms of cardiac disease.*

causes include atrial fibrillation, valvular heart disease, cardiomyopathy, atrial myxoma, and history of myocardial infarct; all of these may predispose to thrombus formation and release of emboli. The patient should be questioned about the presence of these conditions or symptoms consistent with cardiac disease such as shortness of breath, heart palpitations, or chest pain.

Whereas amaurosis fugax is of sudden onset, carotid artery disease may also be associated with other types of transient vision loss of less abrupt onset but of longer duration (Table 16-4). This type of vision loss tends to involve concentric contraction of the visual field rather than a sectoral or altitudinal pattern. Patients will often complain of peculiar visual aberrations including loss of or excess contrast, or flickering

> *Ask about symptoms of chronic carotid disease.*

Table 16–4 Signs and Symptoms of Ocular Hypoperfusion

Symptoms
Transient vision loss of duration longer than amaurosis fugax
Concentric contraction of visual field
Loss of contrast
Excessive contrast
Flickering lights
Unilateral or bilateral vision loss in bright light
Ocular angina
Signs
Hypoperfusion retinopathy
Ocular ischemic syndrome

lights. These patients may also complain of unilateral or bilateral loss of vision when exposed to bright light; this occurs because chronic retinal ischemia leads to an inability of the retina to effectively resynthesize visual pigment. These patients may also have intense pain in and around the eye (ocular angina) due to ischemia of the trigeminal nerve.

Problems not directly related to the carotid arteries may also cause subacute transient vision loss. Poor cardiac output (pump failure) as in congestive heart failure will cause poor blood supply to one or both eyes and cause temporary visual changes. Similar visual symptoms may be seen with poor blood flow due to hyperviscosity or hypercoagulable states. Patients should be questioned about the presence of blood diseases or symptoms such as fatigue, shortness of breath, bruising, or coldness or swelling in the extremities.

Ask about symptoms related to poor blood flow, i.e., CHF, blood dyscrasias.

Brief periods of vision loss may also be seen in association with disc edema or crowded optic nerves. Called transient visual obscurations, these are very rapid periods of blindness lasting seconds or less in one or both eyes and should not be confused with the stereotypical forms of vision loss seen with amaurosis fugax or migraine. Disc edema is the most common cause although other disc conditions, such as disc drusen or congenital anomalies of the optic nerve, may cause them as well.

Some patients may complain of transient vision loss only when the eye is moved into an eccentric position of gaze. Any patient with vision loss associated with eccentric eye position should be suspected of having an orbital mass. The history should try to ascertain whether there is pain on eye movement, noticeable change

Determine if the vision loss is in only one position of gaze.

in the appearance of the eye, or general reduction of vision.

Local ocular conditions such as blepharospasm, tear film abnormalities and ocular surface disease, vitreal debris, or intermittent angle-closure glaucoma can also cause transient visual changes. Dry eye and other diseases of the ocular surface cause visual alterations that fluctuate with blinking, use of artificial tears, and environmental change. Vitreal debris may lead to reports of vision loss when the vitreal opacity passes through the visual axis. The vision loss seen with intermittent angle-closure glaucoma is usually accompanied by halos around lights and pain in and around the eye.

> *Ask about ocular conditions that may cause transient vision loss.*

Primary Actions—History of Transient Vision Loss

- Determine the temporal profile of the event, remembering that migrainous vision loss usually lasts from 15 to 30 minutes, amaurosis fugax from 2 to 15 minutes but usually 3 to 5, and transient visual obscurations on the order of seconds.
- Determine if the vision loss is unilateral or bilateral.
- Determine if there are any accompanying systemic symptoms.
- Determine if the vision loss occurs in an eccentric position of gaze.
- Take a complete medical history to determine the likelihood of a medical (nonmigraine) cause of the vision loss.

EXAMINATION

The eye examination in patients with transient vision loss attempts to discover local ocular signs that might indicate the cause of the vision loss. The clinician should remember that many of the causes of transient vision loss are cerebral in nature and may not be associated with ocular signs. Even when the eye is the primary source of the vision loss, ocular signs are often transitory. The eye examination in most cases of transient vision loss is negative.

In middle-aged and older patients, the most common cause of transient vision loss is ischemia secondary to carotid artery disease. The clinical examination should look for evidence of embolic phenomena or retinal hypoperfusion in these patients.

> *Look for signs of ischemia in older patients with transient vision loss.*

Retinal emboli are often indicative of significant vascular disease (Table 16–5). By far the most commonly observed retinal embolus is the cholesterol

Table 16–5   Retinal Emboli Associated with Vascular Disease

Type	Source	Typical Vision Loss
Cholesterol	Ipsilateral carotid atheroma	None or transient
Platelet-fibrin	Thrombotic material on heart valves or atheroma	None, transient, or arterial occlusion
Calcific	Cardiac valves	Arterial occlusion

embolus, or Hollenhorst plaque (Figure 16–1). Cholesterol emboli made up 87% of visible emboli in one large series. Typically, cholesterol emboli are small, shiny yellow crystals that are lodged at bifurcations, but they sometimes are found in smaller perimacular arterioles or more distal sites. They often appear larger than the retinal vessel they are lodged in. They tend to move distally and disappear from the retinal circulation over the course of hours, days, or weeks. A periarteriolar sheath, a localized inflammatory reaction to the ischemia caused by the embolus, may mark their former presence (Figure 16–2).

Look for retinal emboli.

Cholesterol emboli are presumed to come from ulcerative atheromas of the ipsilateral carotid artery. Those associated with transient vision loss are as-

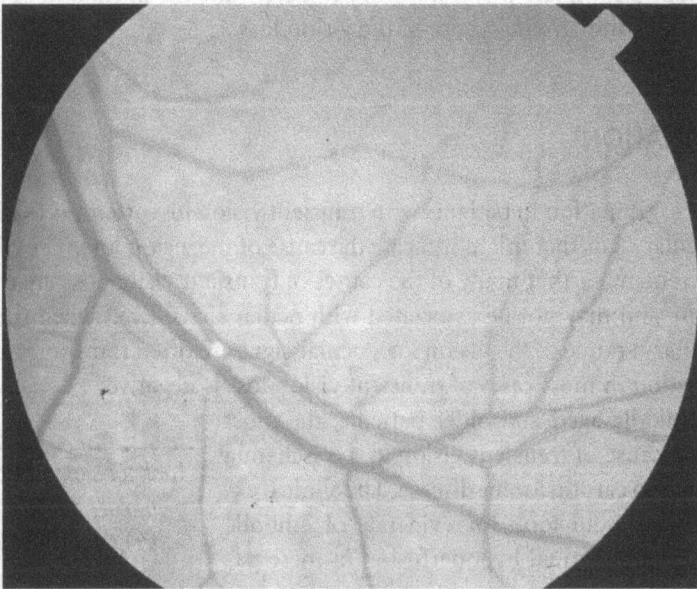

Figure 16–1. Cholesterol embolus lodged at the bifurcation of a retinal arteriole.

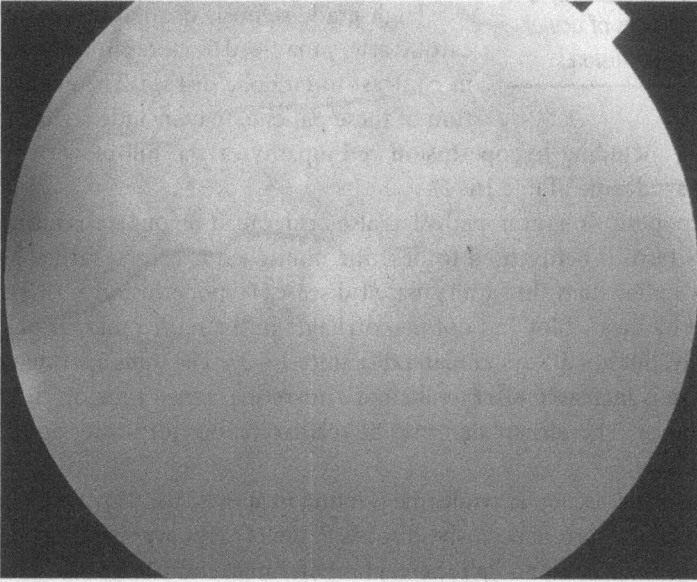

Figure 16–2. Periarteriolar sheath marking the former presence of a cholesterol embolus.

sociated with more active and progressive carotid disease than those that produce no symptoms.

Cholesterol emboli are associated with a decreased survival rate of 13% in the first year after their appearance, 27% at five years, and 40% at the end of eight years.

Platelet-fibrin emboli are the other type of retinal embolus most commonly associated with carotid atherosclerotic disease and transient vision loss. They are grayish-white amorphous masses that tend to jump rapidly from bifurcation to bifurcation fragmenting as they go. Their appearance and migratory behavior make them difficult to observe. They originate from thrombotic material formed on carotid atheromas or from heart valves. They may be associated with no symptoms, transient vision loss, or retinal artery occlusion.

Calcific emboli are single, solid, chalky-white entities lodged in larger arterioles or on the disc itself. They often cause retinal artery occlusion. They are usually not associated with transient vision loss but must be differentiated from cholesterol and platelet-fibrin emboli.

There are other types of retinal emboli that must be differentiated from emboli of vascular origin. Talc from IV drug abuse, fat from release from bone marrow after fracture, tumor material, infectious materials, and IV medications may migrate to the retina and occasionally cause transient vision loss.

*Look for signs of ocular
hypoperfusion.*
High-grade stenosis or total occlusion of the carotid artery may lead to more chronic symptoms in contrast to embolic disease. The eye examination of these patients may include signs of ocular ischemia including hypoperfusion retinopathy or the full-blown ocular ischemic syndrome (Table 16–4).

Hypoperfusion retinopathy has also been called venous stasis retinopathy, but this term is better used to describe nonischemic central retinal vein occlusion rather than this artery-based disease. Hypoperfusion retinopathy is marked by meaty blot and dot hemorrhages in the retinal midperiphery and is usually, but not always, unilateral (Figure 16–3). The veins are often dilated and there is increased artery-vein and arm-retina transit time on fluorescein angiography. The earliest sign may be relative venous tortuosity on the more hypoxic side.

The ocular ischemic syndrome is found in about 5 to 10% of patients with severe bilateral carotid occlusive disease. Patients may have vision ranging anywhere from 20/20 to no light perception and may complain of ischemic pain (ocular angina) in and around the eye from trigeminal nerve ischemia.

Diverse anterior segment signs including conjunctival and episcleral injection, corneal edema, sluggish pupillary response, anterior chamber cells and

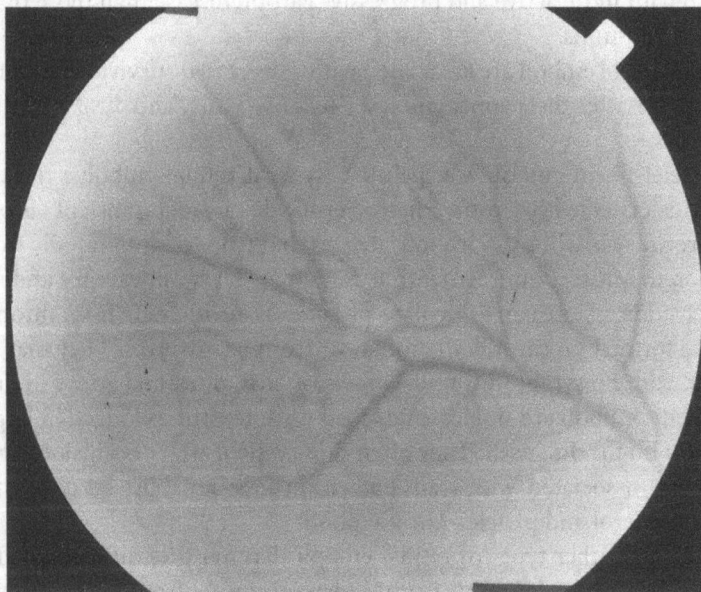

Figure 16–3. Midperipheral dot and blot hemorrhages indicative of hypoperfusion retinopathy.

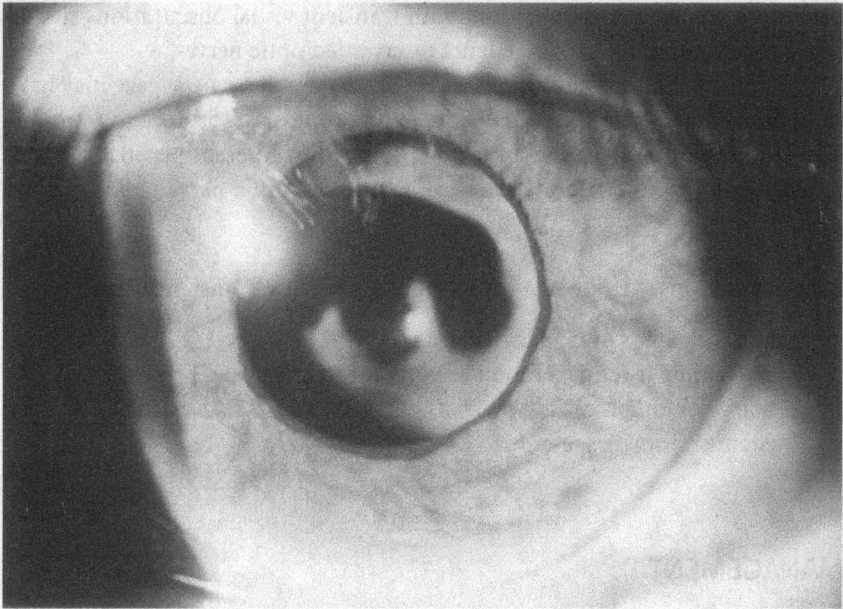

Figure 16–4. Marked iris neovascularization in a patient with the ocular ischemic syndrome. Anterior segment neovascularization is very aggressive when secondary to ocular ischemia and is a very poor prognostic sign.

flare, cataract, and iris and angle neovascularization with neovascular glaucoma may be present (Figure 16–4). The retina will show signs of ischemia including retinal hemorrhages and microaneurysms, cotton-wool spots, changes in vessel caliber, spontaneous arterial pulsations due to low perfusion pressure, and a macular cherry red spot if retinal artery pressure falls below intraocular pressure. Fluorescein angiographic findings will be similar but more severe than seen in hypoperfusion retinopathy including delayed arm-retina and artery-vein transit and patchy choroidal filling.

The presence of the ocular ischemic syndrome indicates very poor ocular perfusion and the clinician should be wary of the development of anterior segment neovascularization that may occur rapidly and progress aggressively. Development of iris or angle neovascularization is a very poor prognostic sign.

The eye examination can rule out other causes of transient vision loss including disc anomalies such as disc edema, disc drusen, intermittent angle-closure glaucoma, blepharospasm, and ocular surface disease, and vitreal or other media opacities.

> *Look for nonischemic ocular signs that may cause transient vision loss.*

Patients with vision loss consistent with transient visual obscurations should be evaluated carefully for disc edema or crowded optic nerves.

Patients with transient vision loss associated with eccentric gaze may have signs of orbital disease: reduced vision, pain, proptosis, resistance to retropulsion, and diplopia; all of these may be progressive. Afferent pupillary defect, reduced color vision, decreased visual acuity, and optic nerve pallor may be seen.

Primary Actions—Examination of the Patient with Transient Vision Loss

- Look for signs of ocular ischemia.
- Determine if retinal emboli are present or have been present.
- Look for other causes of transient vision loss such as dry eye, disc edema/anomalies, etc.

MANAGEMENT

The management of patients with transient vision loss is essentially determining the underlying cause of the vision loss and managing the cause appropriately. As the causes of transient vision loss are usually age-associated, the patient's age should be the initial guide to the work-up (Tables 16–6 and 16–7).

Management of patients with transient vision loss is guided by the patient's age.

Younger patients—those 35 years of age and under—most likely have some form of migraine as the cause of their vision loss. If scintillations are present, or there are other features of classic migraine, the diagnosis is almost certain.

Younger patients are likely to have migraine.

If a migraine diagnosis is questioned, try to determine if the vision loss is monocular or binocular. If it is monocular, retinociliary migraine is likely in the absence of pertinent systemic or ocular findings. Causes of embolic disease in a young patient—mitral valve disease particularly in females, rheumatic heart disease, atrial myxoma, or cardiomyopathy—may also be considered. Consultation with a cardiologist is then indicated.

If the vision loss is monocular but associated with signs and symptoms of an orbital mass, neuro-eye consultation with appropriate neuroimaging (CT, MRI) is indicated (Figure 16–5).

Order neuroimaging when orbital disease is suspected.

Unilateral disc anomalies may also cause

Table 16–6 Management of Younger Patients with Transient Vision Loss

- Is it migraine or is it something else?
  - ○ Are scintillations present?
  - ○ Are other features of "classic" migraine present?
  - ○ If the answer is yes to these 2 questions, then the diagnosis of migraine is almost certain.
- If scintillations are not present, try to determine if the vision loss is monocular or binocular.
  - ○ If binocular, migraine is the likely diagnosis.
    - ■ Increased intracranial pressure, bilateral crowded discs, systemic hematological problems, cardiac insufficiency, and vertebrobasilar insufficiency should be considered.
  - ○ If monocular and lasting for about 5 minutes, retinociliary migraine is the most likely diagnosis.
- Local causes of TVL should be excluded via an eye exam.
- If uncertainty still exists, a general medical exam should be requested to exclude hypertension, hyperviscosity, vasculitis, and hypercoagulability. Mitral valve prolapse, rheumatic heart disease, and atrial myxoma may need to be ruled out as well.
- If all is negative, reassurance and follow-up is generally the best course of action as a search for other causes, i.e., carotid artery disease, will likely prove fruitless.

Table 16–7 Management of Older Patients with Transient Vision Loss

- Is it vascular or is it something else?
- Is the vision loss monocular or binocular?
  - ○ If binocular, are there other signs and symptoms of vertebrobasilar insufficiency? Are there signs of cardiac insufficiency? Could this be migraine in an older patient?
  - ○ If monocular, is it typical of amaurosis fugax?
    - ■ If the vision loss is typical of amaurosis fugax, suspect embolic disease.
    - ■ If the vision loss is monocular but of slower onset and longer duration than amaurosis fugax, suspect ocular hypoperfusion due to carotid or cardiac insufficiency.
- Perform a thorough eye examination to search for retinal emboli, vascular occlusions, and signs of poor perfusion.
- A cardiology consult is indicated to rule out cardiac sources of emboli and generalized cardiac disease.
- The carotid system should be evaluated noninvasively by duplex scanning and MRA. The results of the noninvasive testing will guide the follow-up: do nothing, treat medically, or order invasive testing and consider surgical treatment.

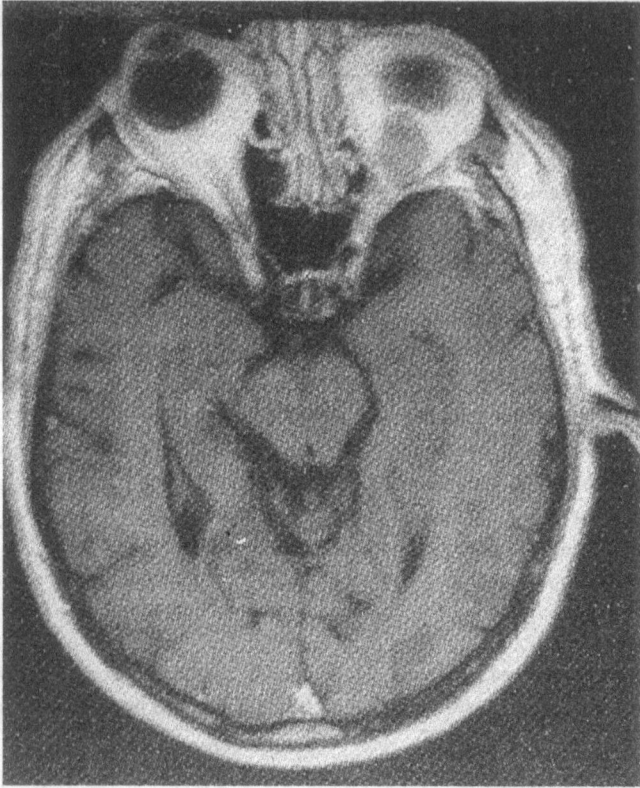

Figure 16–5. MRI showing orbital mass causing compression of the optic nerve and proptosis.

monocular transient vision loss. Sequential disc photos and visual fields to document progression should be used to manage these patients. The clinician should remember that disc drusen are not benign and can cause progressive visual field loss.

If the vision loss is binocular, migraine is the likely diagnosis, but bilateral crowded discs, blood dyscrasia, vertebrobasilar disease, and cardiac insufficiency must be considered. Patients who have disc edema must be evaluated by consultation with a neuro-eye specialist with appropriate neuroimaging. Lumbar puncture is indicated when increased intracranial pressure or infection is suspected. Consultation with an internist to rule out hyperviscosity syndromes (e.g., polycythemia, leukemia, thrombocytopenia, macroglobulinemia, multiple myeloma), hypercoagulability (e.g., protein S or protein C deficiency, antiphospholipid antibody syndrome), or vasculitis may be indicated. CBC with differential, ESR, tests of coagulation, antiphospholipid anti-

Table 16–8 Hyperviscosity, Hypercoagulability, and Vasculitic
Conditions Associated with Transient Vision Loss

Hyperviscosity and hypercoagulability
  Leukemia
  Polycythemia
  Thrombocytopenia
  Paraproteinemia
    Multiple myeloma
    Macroglobulinemia
  Abnormal platelet aggregability
    Protein S deficiency
    Protein C deficiency
    Antithrombin III deficiency
  Antiphospholipid antibody syndrome
    Lupus anticoagulant
    Anticardiolipin antibody
  Disseminated intravascular coagulopathy (DIC)
  Inflammatory bowel disease
  Migraine
  Oral contraceptive use
Vasculitis
    Systemic lupus erythematosus (SLE) and other collagen vascular diseases
    Sarcoidosis
    Giant cell arteritis
    Takayasu disease
    Polyarteritis nodosa
    Syphilis
    Lyme disease
    Infectious meningitis

bodies, and tests for specific causes of vasculitis, e.g., syphilis, may need to be ordered (Table 16–8).

The older patient with transient vision loss—aged 45 or older—should be considered to have a vascular etiology until proven otherwise. Athero-sclerotic disease is usually the underlying etiology.

Older patients should be considered as having a vascular cause of their vision loss.

The determination of monocular versus binocular vision loss is crucial.

If the vision loss is truly binocular, other signs of vertebrobasilar insufficiency or cardiac insufficiency should be sought to explain the loss of vision. The clinician must wonder if migraine is a potential diagnosis, keeping in mind that the diagnosis of new-onset migraine in an older patient is fraught with danger.

Table 16–9   Carotid and Cardiac Evaluation of Patients with Transient Vision Loss

Carotid evaluation
  Noninvasive
    Duplex scanning
    Magnetic resonance angiography (MRA)
  Invasive
    Angiography
Cardiac evaluation
  EKG
  Holter monitor
  Echocardiography
    Transthoracic (TTE)—noninvasive
    Transesophageal (TEE)—invasive

Patients with suspected vertebrobasilar insufficiency require noninvasive vascular workup, specifically MRA. Significant vertebrobasilar disease should be managed medically as surgical treatment has been shown to be ineffective (see below). Cardiac workup includes EKG, Holter monitor, and echocardiography (see below).

If the vision loss is monocular and consistent with amaurosis fugax, the patient should be evaluated for atherosclerosis with particular attention paid to the carotid arteries and heart (Table 16–9). Co-management with an internist is indicated. Presence of hypertension, diabetes, smoking, alcohol abuse, use of estrogen in women, and family history of cardiovascular disease must be elicited, as these factors are associated with atherosclerotic disease. Blood pressure, blood glucose, a complete blood count, and a lipid profile are minimal office and laboratory studies to be undertaken.

Examine the heart and carotid arteries in patients with amaurosis fugax.

In-office palpation and auscultation of the carotids to discern carotid pulse or the presence of carotid bruit and/or ophthalmodynamometry to evaluate retinal perfusion pressure is not necessary as it is not likely to change the management of the case. Our feeling is that if you need to feel or listen to the carotids, the patient should have noninvasive carotid evaluation.

The noninvasive assessment of the patient's carotid system usually begins with carotid duplex scanning. The duplex scan combines B-mode ultrasound with pulsed Doppler imaging to produce a dynamic picture of the anatomy of the blood vessel and blood flow through it (Figure 16–6). Degree of stenosis can be easily calculated and shows a high correlation with cerebral angiogra-

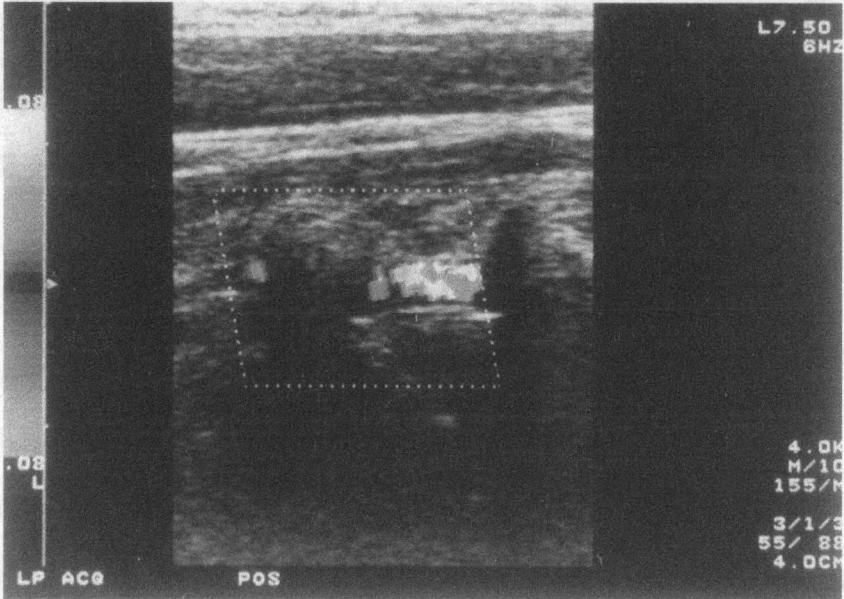

Figure 16–6. Duplex scan of the internal carotid artery. Velocity and direction of blood flow are color-coded.

phy although the differentiation between very high degrees of stenosis and complete vessel occlusion is not always clear. Plaque morphology—calcification, hemorrhage—and plaque ulceration are shown particularly well by this technique. A very important caveat is that this procedure is highly technician-driven and accurate results are dependent upon the skill and experience of the person doing the testing. Carotid duplex scanning remains an inexpensive, noninvasive, accurate way to evaluate both degree of stenosis and presence of plaque ulceration or hemorrhage.

Over the last 10 years, another technique to noninvasively evaluate the cerebral circulation has been developed. Magnetic resonance angiography (MRA) is essentially MRI of moving blood (Figure 16–7). MRA has the distinct advantage of being able to evaluate not only the extracranial carotid system but also the intracranial vessels without the need for the injection of contrast material. As the technique has evolved and improved, it now shows good correlation with angiography. MRA is not as effective as carotid duplex scanning in assessing plaque morphology or ulceration. MRA is also more expensive than duplex scanning as it is usually done in conjunction with a full MRI study. Contraindications to MRA are the same as those to MRI—retained metallic foreign bodies, aneurysm clips, and cardiac pacemakers.

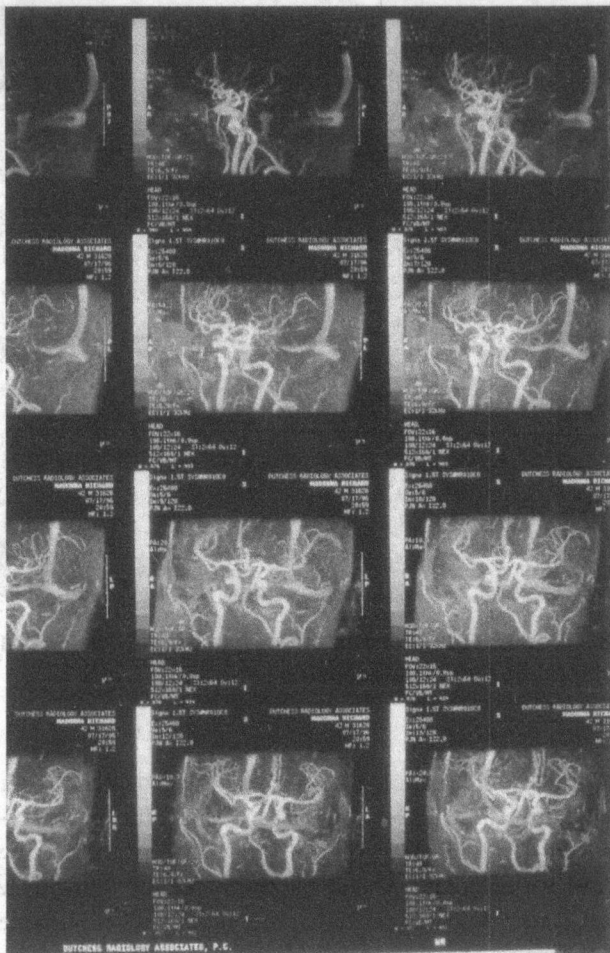

Figure 16–7. MRA of the extracranial and intracranial circulation. MRA is able to image this circulation without the injection of contrast material.

The use of carotid duplex scanning and MRA in tandem to evaluate plaque morphology, plaque ulceration, and degree of stenosis of both the extracranial and intracranial circulation has obviated the need for angiography and its associated morbidity and mortality in some patients.

The so-called "gold standard" for evaluation of the extracranial and intracranial circulation is cerebral angiography (Figure 16–8). Angiography involves the injection of a radiopaque dye into a catheter that has been threaded into the femoral artery, up into the abdominal aorta, around the heart, and into the arch of the aorta. From there, dye can be selectively released into each

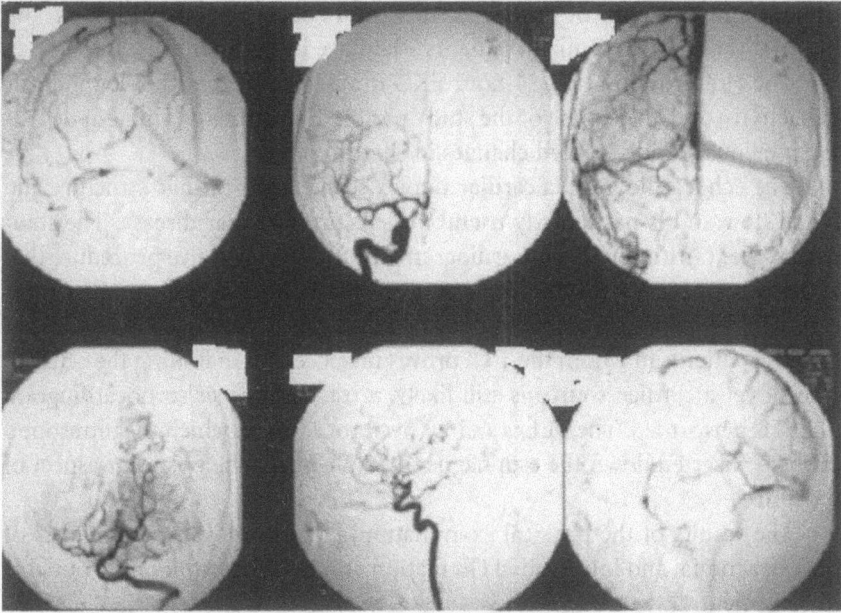

Figure 16–8.   Cerebral angiography of the extracranial and intracranial circulation. Detail is best with angiography but risks include stroke and myocardial infarct.

of the four major vessels that supply the brain: the left and right common carotid arteries and the left and right vertebral arteries. Vessel stenosis/occlusion and blood flow are exquisitely shown.

   Unfortunately, angiography is not without risks. Morbidity in the form of stroke and myocardial infarct and mortality are not uncommon. Because of this risk, angiography is normally reserved for those patients who are surgical candidates, those who have unexplained symptoms, or those who may be harboring intracerebral vascular lesions such as aneurysms or arteriovenous malformations.

> *Remember the risk of angiography when advising patients.*

   As stated above, the need for angiography has been reduced by improvements in duplex scanning and MRA. Some institutions will use a combination of duplex scanning and MRA in place of angiography in some patients.

   The heart must be evaluated not only as a source of emboli but also because patients with amaurosis fugax and carotid artery disease have generalized atherosclerotic disease that is likely to affect the heart.

   An electrocardiogram (EKG) is essential for evaluation of the heart's rhythm and detection of problems such as previous myocardial infarct, but may not detect arrhythmia in patients who have intermittent disease.

The Holter monitor, a 24-hour EKG done in concert with a log indicating activity over the course of the study period, may prove essential in detecting previously undiscovered changes in rhythm.

The echocardiogram, a cardiac duplex scan, shows cardiac structure and blood flow and is particularly useful in detecting valvular disease. The standard is the transthoracic echocardiogram (TTE), a noninvasive procedure that is performed by placing the ultrasound probe beside the sternum. In most cases, TTE is sufficiently able to detect cardiac causes of transient vision loss. In those patients in whom the TTE proves unsuccessful in finding the cause of disease yet a cardiac source is still likely, a transesophageal echocardiogram (TEE) is performed. The TEE is an invasive procedure in which the ultrasound probe is inserted down the esophagus to better image the posterior aspect of the heart.

The results of the physical examination, laboratory tests, and studies of the extracranial and intracranial circulation and heart determine the course of management.

Patients with significant carotid artery disease are candidates for carotid endarterectomy. Appropriate use of this surgery in patients with transient vision loss has been guided by studies in the 1990s, particularly the North American Symptomatic Carotid Endarterectomy Trial (NASCET). The NASCET study showed that in patients with transient ischemic attack (including amaurosis fugax) or mild stroke, carotid endarterectomy significantly reduced future stroke risk in those patients with 70% or greater carotid artery stenosis. When the data were further evaluated, patients with amaurosis fugax and greater than 70% carotid stenosis were shown to have an 8% per year risk of stroke as opposed to the 2% risk reported historically for patients with amaurosis. This study showed that patients with amaurosis fugax alone might be candidates for carotid endarterectomy. Despite these results, the clinician should always remember that this procedure still carries a significant morbidity and mortality risk, and that each case should be handled on an individual basis in consultation with a neurosurgeon.

Nonsurgical candidates with significant atherosclerotic disease need to be managed medically by their internist or cardiologist. Aspirin (acetylsalicylic acid, ASA) has been the traditional treatment for these patients. Doses as low as 30 mg are effective in significantly reducing platelet aggregation, thereby reducing stroke risk. A single baby aspirin per day (81 mg) is usually an appropriate dose. The risks of aspirin therapy such as gastrointestinal bleeding and discomfort and generalized increases in clotting time should not be forgotten.

More powerful platelet antiaggregants are available for those patients intolerant to ASA or in whom aspirin is ineffective. Ticlopidine, which works directly on the platelet cell membrane, has been shown to reduce stroke risk more than ASA in patients with TIA but at much greater cost and with increased side effects such as GI upset. Clopidogrel is a newer drug with similar efficacy as compared to ticlopidine with fewer side effects.

Cardiac problems causing transient vision loss should be comanaged with a cardiologist. The spectrum of disease includes arrhythmia, valvular disease, myocardial infarct, and cardiomyopathy. Management includes medication to control heart rhythm and improve circulation, surgery such as cardiac pacemaker implantation, or both.

A neurologist or other physician skilled in the treatment of the condition should manage migraine. Treatment approaches include medication (beta-blockers, antidepressants, analgesics, medications specific to migraine), biofeedback, and avoidance of migraine triggers.

> *Refer to a neurologist for care of migraine.*

Depending on the cause, an internist, hematologist, oncologist, or rheumatologist manages hypercoagulability and hyperviscosity states. Treatment of the underlying cause of the problem will usually reduce the incidence of transient vision loss.

Primary Actions—Management of Transient Vision Loss

- Determine the cause of the transient vision loss. The age of the patient will guide the workup.
- Suspect migraine in the younger patient.
- Suspect vascular disease in the older patient.
- Manage the patient based on the cause of the vision loss. Many patients require comanagement with a neurologist, internist, cardiologist, or vascular surgeon.
- Stay abreast of major developments in the management of conditions pertinent to transient vision loss to better guide your patients.

Chapter 17

Acute, Persistent Vision Loss

"Doctor, I suddenly lost the vision in my eye and it hasn't come back."

SCOPE OF THE PROBLEM

There are few things as traumatic as sudden loss of vision. Often, the vision loss is a manifestation of an underlying systemic condition that requires follow-up care. The optometrist must provide acute care for the vision loss and also manage the systemic condition with other practitioners. Many patients often delay seeking care in the hope that their vision will return. This delay will sometimes prevent them from getting treatment that might have reversed some or all of their blindness. Unfortunately, in many cases no treatment exists and the practitioner is left only to try to discover the cause of the vision loss and hopefully prevent it from occurring in the opposite eye.

HISTORY

Description of the Event

The history should attempt to elicit laterality and the time course of the vision loss. The patient should be asked which eye was affected and how the vision loss was noticed. Sudden, bilateral vision loss is extremely rare and when it is reported it is often because the patient has suddenly lost vision

Establish laterality, time course, tempo, quantity, and how the vision loss was noticed.

in the eye opposite one that previously had poor vision. The patient should be questioned as to how suddenly the vision was lost (instantaneously vs. over the course of minutes or hours), to describe the tempo of the loss (immediate and

Obtain a medical and ocular history to uncover risk factors for vision loss. complete vs. gradual), and whether the whole field or part of the field was involved. The presence or absence of pain should be elicited as well. Clear answers to these questions along with known risk factors such as age, medical history, and previous ocular history should narrow the list of differentials.

Patients Older than Age 50

Sudden vision loss in an older individual (Table 17–1) is associated with a myriad of causes including optic nerve disease, macular disease, and retinal disease.

Optic Nerve Disease

Optic neuropathies in this age group are typically ischemic in nature. In most cases, patients will report acute onset of vision loss. Occasionally, nonarteritic anterior ischemic optic neuropathy (NAION) will progress after an acute onset of relatively milder vision loss. Nonarteritic ischemic optic neuropathy occurs without accompanying systemic symptoms. Patients will often have a history of vascular disease.

Patients older than age 65 should be suspected as having giant cell arteritis and must be evaluated for this condition. These patients may describe

Table 17–1 Common Causes of Acute, Persistent Vision Loss in Older Patients

Optic nerve disease
   Nonarteritic anterior ischemic optic neuropathy (NAION)
   Arteritic anterior ischemic optic neuropathy (AAION)
Macular disease
   Exudative age-related macular degeneration (wet AMD)
Retinal disease
   Central retinal artery occlusion (CRAO)
   Branch retinal artery occlusion (BRAO)
   Central retinal vein occlusion (CRVO)
   Branch retinal vein occlusion (BRVO)
Retinal detachment
Media opacification
   Vitreous hemorrhage
   Corneal decompensation
   Uveitis

headache, jaw claudication, neck pain, weight loss, fever, and malaise in association with the loss of vision. However, it should always be remembered that arteritic anterior ischemic optic neuropathy (AAION) could occur without accompanying signs or symptoms.

> *If AAION is suspected, ask about symptoms associated with giant cell arteritis.*

Macular Disease

Sudden, central vision loss in the older patient is most frequently associated with exudative age-related macular degeneration (AMD). Established patients will likely have a history of dry AMD noted in their charts. A family history of AMD may be present but it is not a terribly useful finding as the clinical appearance of AMD is usually clear-cut. Patients with exudative AMD are usually Caucasian; those with light-colored irides are at greatest risk. Smok-

> *Ask about risk factors for AMD.*

ing, vascular disease, ultraviolet light exposure, and a variety of nutritional deficiencies are also associated.

Retinal Vascular Occlusive Disease

Sudden, persistent vision loss associated with retinal vascular occlusive disease may be minimal or profound depending on the type and location of the occlusion. Systemic cardiovascular disease is

> *Ask about previous bouts of transient vision loss.*

often noted in these patients. A history of transient vision loss preceding the attack should be sought (see Chapter 16).

Central retinal artery occlusion (CRAO) is associated with severe, sudden, painless vision loss. Central retinal vein occlusion (CRVO) is also associated with severe vision loss, but this vision loss is often not as profound as with central artery occlusion.

Branch retinal artery occlusions (BRAO) and vein occlusions (BRVO) affect central vision if the macular vessels are involved. If the macular region is not involved, patients may notice a loss of the visual field that corresponds to the portion of the retina affected by the occlusion or they may be asymptomatic.

Retinal Detachment

Rhegmatogenous retinal detachment may cause relatively sudden vision loss if the patient notices the associated field defect or if the macula is involved. An abrupt increase in floaters and the ap-

> *Ask about sudden onset of numerous floaters and photopsia if RD is suspected.*

pearance of photopsia are often associated (see Chapter 18). A history of myopia, previous cataract surgery, or vitreoretinal disease, especially lattice degeneration, may be present.

Media Opacification

Sudden loss of media clarity is most commonly due to vitreous hemorrhage but may also be due to corneal decompensation or anterior or posterior chamber inflammation. Vitreous hemorrhage is seen most commonly in patients with proliferative retinopathies. Occasionally, patients may have a dense cataract that they had not noticed until they covered the better-seeing eye.

Patients Younger than Age 40

Younger patients with sudden vision loss (Table 17–2) are more of a challenge because the number of potential etiologies goes well beyond those related to cardiovascular disease. The incidence of vascular disease is much lower, so ischemic optic neuropathy and vascular occlusions occur much less commonly. The risk of nontraumatic retinal detachment is also lower. Central vision loss due to age-related macular degeneration is not an issue but choroidal neovascularization from other causes may occur.

Table 17–2 Common Causes of Acute, Persistent Vision Loss in Younger Patients

Optic nerve disease
  Optic neuritis
  Inflammatory disorders
  Infectious disorders
  Toxic disorders
  Metabolic disorders
  Hereditary disorders
  Other
Macular disease
  Choroidal neovascularization
    High myopia
    Angioid streaks
    Ocular histoplasmosis
    Multifocal choroiditis
    Idiopathic
    Other
Retinal detachment

Optic Nerve Disease

Sudden, unilateral vision loss in a patient aged 20 to 50 years in association with pain on eye movement is characteristic of optic neuritis. In typical optic neuritis, patients will have reduced visual acuity, color vision, and contrast sensitivity that will stabilize at about 14 days. An improvement in visual function is expected after this time. Pain on eye movements is highly characteristic and may help separate optic neuritis from other optic neuropathies, particularly ischemic optic neuropathy. A previous history of multiple sclerosis may be

> *Ask about pain on eye movements, weakness, numbness, urinary incontinence, and Uhthoff's phenomenon.*

present, the patient may complain of neurological symptoms including weakness, numbness, urinary incontinence, or Uhthoff's phenomenon, or the vision loss may occur in isolation. Optic neuritis may be a forme fruste of multiple sclerosis or it may be the first indicator of the impending development of the disease.

Other optic neuropathies also must be considered in this age group. Vision loss seen in the non-optic neuritis group may present quite similarly to optic neuritis, although usually without pain. The tempo of the vision loss will be less acute than in typical optic neuritis and vision recovery will be less predictable or will not occur at all. The practitioner should carefully seek a history of traumatic, inflammatory, infectious, toxic, metabolic, or other systemic disease. Sarcoidosis, syphilis, Lyme disease, or chronic alcoholism occurs most commonly. A family history of

> *Ask about history of traumatic, inflammatory, infectious, toxic, metabolic, or other systemic disease.*

blindness should also be investigated as some forms of hereditary optic nerve disease may present in this age group. In the last few years it has become clear that the genetic mutations causing Leber's hereditary optic neuropathy are much more common than previously thought.

Macular Disease

Besides AMD, choroidal neovascularization may develop in association with a myriad of other causes that may affect younger persons. These include, but are not limited to, pathological myopia, angioid streaks, ocular histoplasmosis, multifocal choroiditis, and idiopathic causes. The history should include a search for clues to associated systemic conditions including collagen or elastic tissue disease (pseudoxanthoma

> *Ask about personal characteristics or conditions associated with choroidal neovascularization.*

elasticum) or living in an area endemic for histoplasmosis such as river valleys.

Macular dystrophies such as Stargardt's disease or Best's disease will cause central vision loss but these patients do not present acutely.

Retinal Detachment

The complaints of younger patients with rhegmatogenous retinal detachment are the same as those of older patients. History of high myopia and vitreoretinal disease may have been previously documented.

Pediatric Patients

Sudden vision loss in the very young is usually associated with congenital or hereditary causes or with trauma. A search for a family history of vision loss at a young age is essential. Concomitant genetic disease or other developmental abnormality is often present. The evaluation of these patients is beyond the scope of this book.

Primary Actions—History of Permanent Vision Loss

- Have the patient describe the vision loss and be sure to answer the questions of laterality, onset, severity, duration, frequency, and progression.
- Tailor the history toward the most likely cause of the vision loss; e.g., ask about pain on eye movement in the younger patient or symptoms of GCA in the older patient.

EXAMINATION

Patients with acute, persistent vision loss will almost always have eye examination findings that give clues to the etiology of the problem. Diseases of the retina and optic nerve are much more common than sudden loss of media clarity. The clinician should keep in mind that although the patient may report sudden vision loss, it is possible that the examination may reveal decreased vision due to a nonacute problem such as a cataract. Patients may discover a problem such as this only because of accidental covering of the better-seeing eye.

Visual Function

Visual acuity should be measured with current spectacles and with a pinhole. A refraction to determine best corrected vision may be helpful if there is any question about the presence or extent of the vision change. Visual acuity may be near-normal in some patients who report sudden vision loss; the patient may be reporting change in color perception or contrast sensitivity.

Establish best corrected visual acuity.

Assessment of color perception is useful in separating optic nerve disease from other causes of vision loss. Red cap desaturation or decreased color vision tested with Ishihara plates is usually a good indicator of optic nerve disease. Reduced

Measure color vision, brightness sense, and contrast sensitivity.

brightness sense is also a good indicator of afferent pathway disease. Contrast sensitivity testing will be reduced in optic nerve disease but is also affected by media opacity and macular disease.

Visual field testing will reveal the extent of vision loss. Confrontation visual field testing via finger counting or with more sensitive targets such as small lights or red targets can be very accurate in plotting out field loss. Amsler grid testing can plot the central 20 degrees and discern whether central field loss is relative or absolute or is associated with metamorphopsia. Goldmann visual fields or automated perimetry can better quantify field loss at

Measure the extent and sensitivity of the visual field.

the expense of examination time. The more time-consuming tests can sometimes be delayed until a definitive diagnosis is established.

Objective tests such as the visual evoked potential (VEP) or electroretinogram (ERG) are excellent in patients who cannot provide appropriate responses to other measures of visual function, in those whose diagnosis is questionable by other measures, in those with suspected pathway disorders (VEP) or with generalized retinal disease (ERG), or in suspected malingerers (VEP).

Extraocular Motilities

Pain on eye movement is highly suggestive of inflammatory disease affecting the optic nerve, particularly optic neuritis. In the context of acute, persistent vision loss, restriction of motility may be associated with a retrobulbar mass compressing the optic nerve, thyroid orbitopathy, orbital pseudotumor, or intracerebral abnormality affecting the

Assess EOMs.

visual pathway as well as the cranial nerves. Sudden vision loss is not as common as slowly progressive loss in these patients.

Pupillary Examination

Careful pupillary examination is essential in the examination of these patients. Presence of an afferent pupillary defect usually indicates optic nerve disease although extensive retinal disease (CRAO, retinal detachment) or macular disease is possible. An attempt to quantify the degree of the afferent defect should be made. Even in the absence of a frank afferent defect, measurement of the size of the pupils in light and dark and their level of reactivity may prove useful in establishing a diagnosis or for future reference.

> *Carefully assess pupillary function.*

Slit Lamp Examination

Slit lamp examination will reveal whether the media is clear and may reveal other clues to the cause of the vision loss. Sudden onset of loss of media clarity is associated with acute hydrops in keratoconus or subacute corneal decompensation as in Fuch's dystrophy or after anterior segment surgery. Again, unilateral cataract may be perceived as causing sudden loss of vision in those patients who accidentally cover the noncataractous eye. The presence of iris or angle neovascularization in a patient with sudden vision loss indicates posterior segment ischemia. Anterior segment neovascularization is most often due to diabetic retinopathy, retinal vein occlusion, retinal artery occlusion, or ocular ischemia. Its presence in a patient with vitreous hemorrhage can prove very useful in determining a cause. Loss of media clarity due to vitreous hemorrhage or vitritis is better evaluated as part of the examination of the posterior pole.

> *Perform a slit lamp examination.*

Tonometry

Markedly elevated IOP may be a sign of acute angle-closure glaucoma or neovascular glaucoma, or may be associated with corneal decompensation. Abnormally low IOP may be an indicator of retinal detachment, ocular ischemia, ocular inflammation, or acute retinal vein occlusion.

> *Measure IOP.*

Posterior Pole Examination

Careful examination of the posterior pole will provide the highest yield in the examination of these patients.

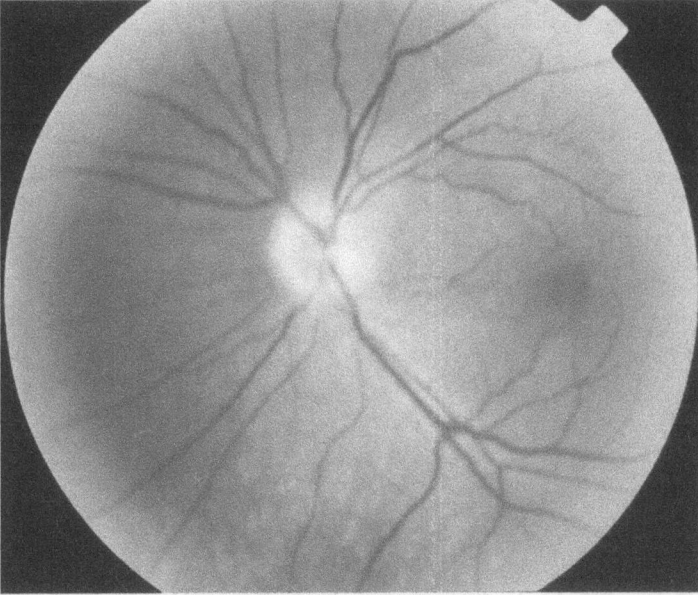

Figure 17–1. Swollen optic nerve head (papillitis) in a young woman with multiple sclerosis.

Poor view of the fundus is an indicator of loss of media clarity from the causes listed previously. The presence of vitreous hemorrhage or vitritis can be ascertained through binocular indirect ophthalmoscopic examination or use of the fundus contact lenses at the slit lamp. If the fundus cannot be visualized, B-scan ultra-sonography should be performed to determine whether the retina is attached and whether there is blood in the vitreous.

> *Perform a dilated fundus examination.*

Acute optic neuritis may be accompanied by hyperemia and edema of the nerve head (papillitis) (Figure 17–1). However, about two-thirds of patients with typical optic neuritis will have inflammation of the postlaminar optic nerve (retrobulbar optic neuritis); their optic nerve heads will appear normal. In ischemic optic neuropathy the optic nerve will appear swollen, often at one pole. Arteritic ischemic optic neuropathy will sometimes appear as a white, swollen nerve head ("pale edema") while nonarteritic ischemic optic neuropathy is associated with a hyperemic nerve (Figure 17–2).

Choroidal neovascularization will appear as macular edema, blood, exudate, or as a discoloration in the central retina (Figure 17–3). In AMD, patients will commonly have drusen and RPE change that may be easier to see

A

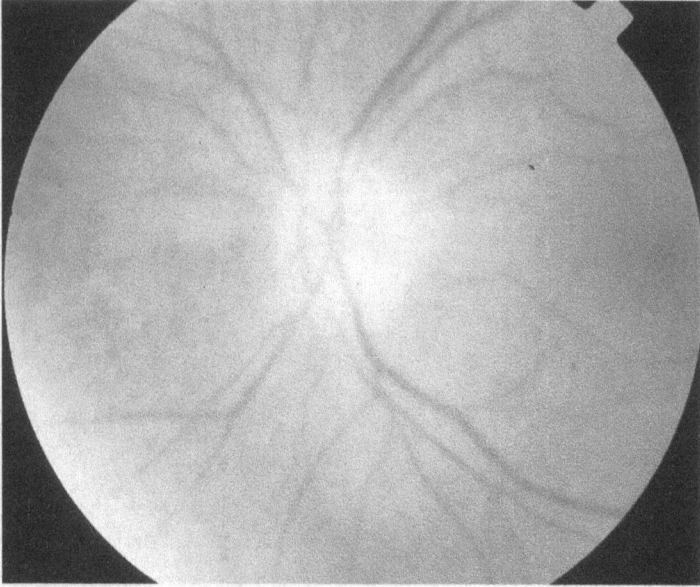

B

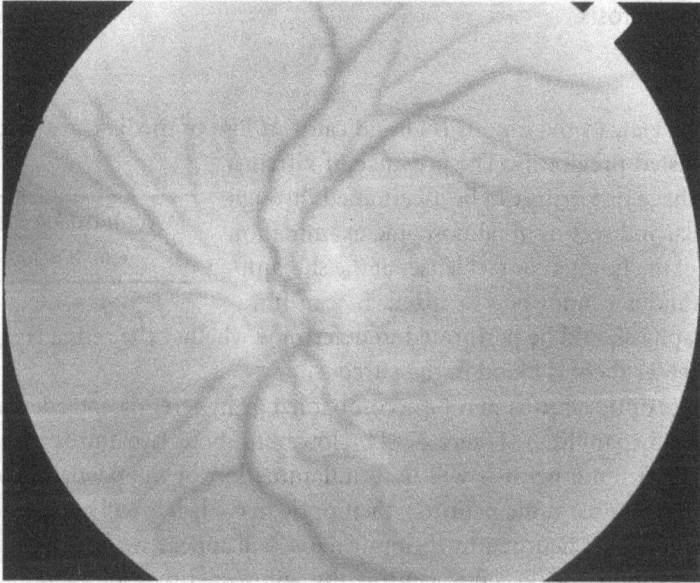

Figure 17–2. (A) "Pale edema" of a patient with AAION. The patient had visual acuity of 20/80 but a markedly constricted visual field. (B) A hyperemic, edematous disc of a patient with NAION.

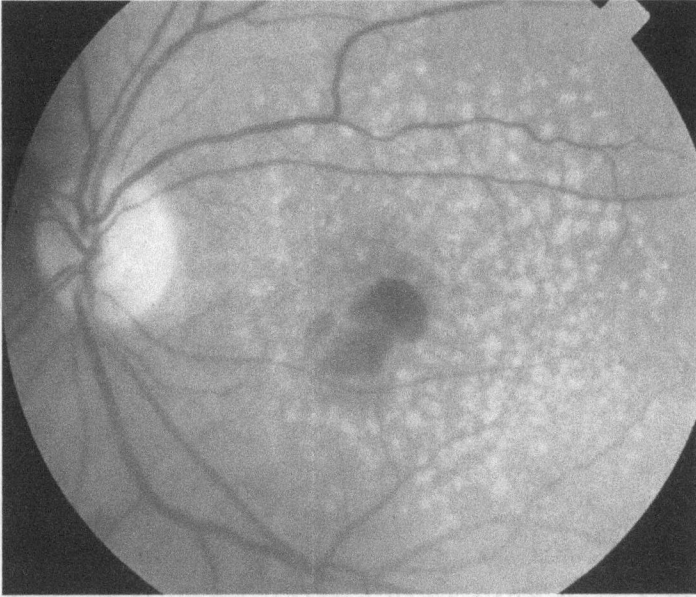

Figure 17–3. A hemorrhagic and edematous macula from an underlying choroidal neovascular membrane.

in the opposite eye. Some of these patients will have disciform scars from wet AMD in the opposite eye. The actual membrane is often difficult to see although a gray-green membrane may be visible. The clinician should remember that choroidal neovascularization may be very subtle and should be suspected in any patient at high risk for the condition, such as those with drusen, RPE changes, histoplasmosis, or angioid streaks, and in any patient who reports sudden change in central vision or in the Amsler grid.

Acute CRAO appears as pale, edematous retina with a macular cherry red spot (Figure 17–4). A patent cilioretinal artery will spare the portion of the retina that it subserves. A calcific embolus may be present at the disc at the site of the occlusion although a visible embolus is not always present. It should be remembered that not all cases of CRAO are embolic in nature; inflammatory, infectious, and other causes are well known. BRAO will have a similar retinal appearance as CRAO in the territory of the branch artery (Figure 17–5). A visible embolus composed of cholesterol, platelet-fibrin material, or calcium will likely be present.

Acute CRVO has tortuous, dilated veins in all four quadrants with intraretinal hemorrhage and edema. Nonischemic and ischemic varieties have been described. Generally, the extent and severity of the fundus involvement are correlated with the level of ischemia (Figure 17–6). Large amounts of

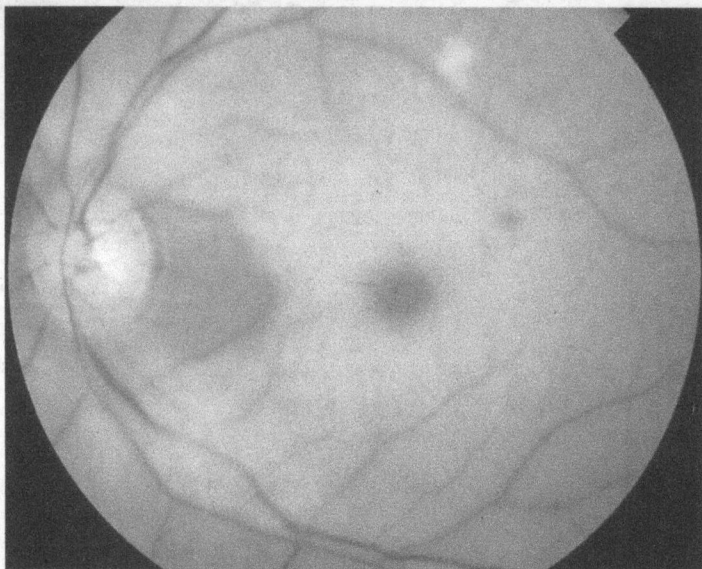

Figure 17–4.   Acute CRAO in a 60-year-old male patient with significant vascular disease. Note the small area of perfused retina from a patent cilioretinal artery.

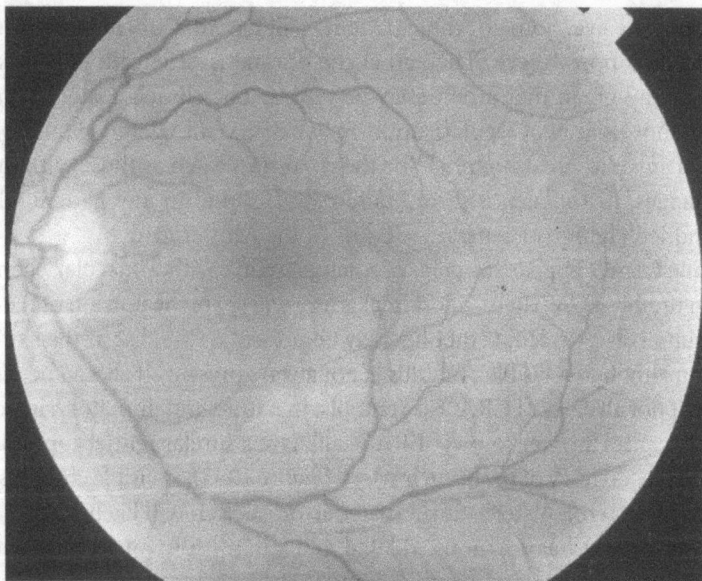

Figure 17–5.   Acute BRAO in a 70-year-old male patient. Note the visible embolus lodged at the arteriolar bifurcation.

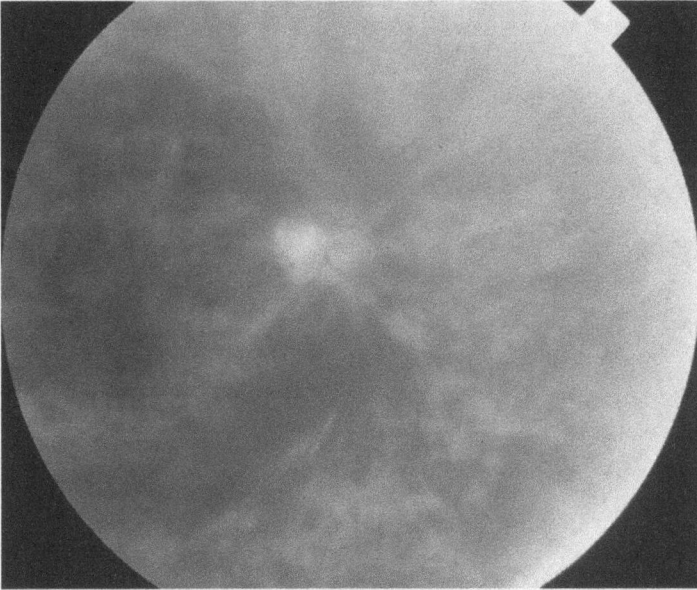

Figure 17–6. This 81-year-old male patient presented with a sudden onset of decreased vision. VA of 20/400 combined with a 2+ relative afferent pupillary defect indicated that the CRVO was likely ischemic.

intraretinal hemorrhage, visual acuity worse than 20/200, and an afferent pupillary defect are highly correlated with ischemia. Ischemic CRVOs have the potential to cause anterior segment neovascularization. BRVO has intraretinal hemorrhage and edema in the distribution of the occluded vessel. The occlusion will be at an arteriovenous crossing (Figure 17–7). Larger BRVOs are associated with ischemia and the potential for disc or retinal neovascularization.

Acute retinal detachment is identified by an elevated retina that billows on eye movement (Figure 17–8). The clinician should search for retinal breaks as a cause of the detachment. Of utmost importance is making the determination of whether the macula is on or off as this is critical in determining the rapidity in which treatment is needed.

Primary Actions—Examination of the Patient with Persistent Vision Loss

- A thorough eye examination will usually reveal the source of the vision loss in these patients.
- The fundus examination has the highest yield in determining the etiology of persistent vision loss.

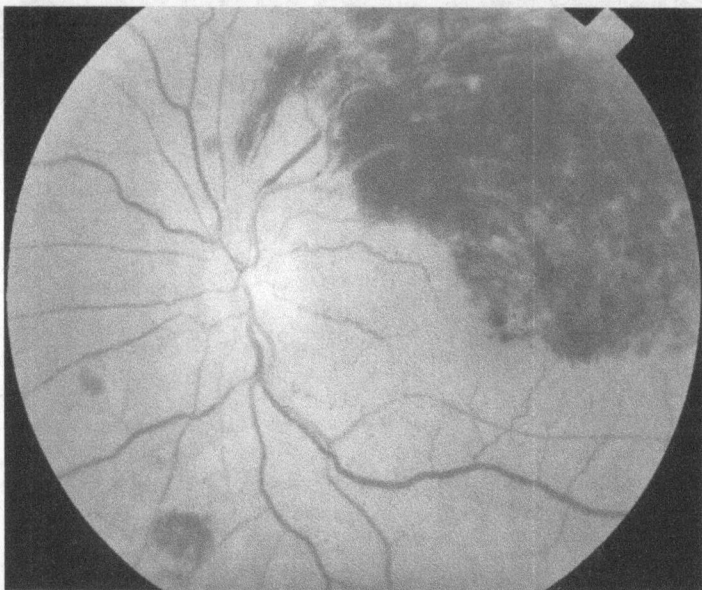

Figure 17–7. A classic BRVO at the first arteriovenous crossing. There is extensive intraretinal hemorrhage and edema extending into the macula. Visual acuity is 20/80.

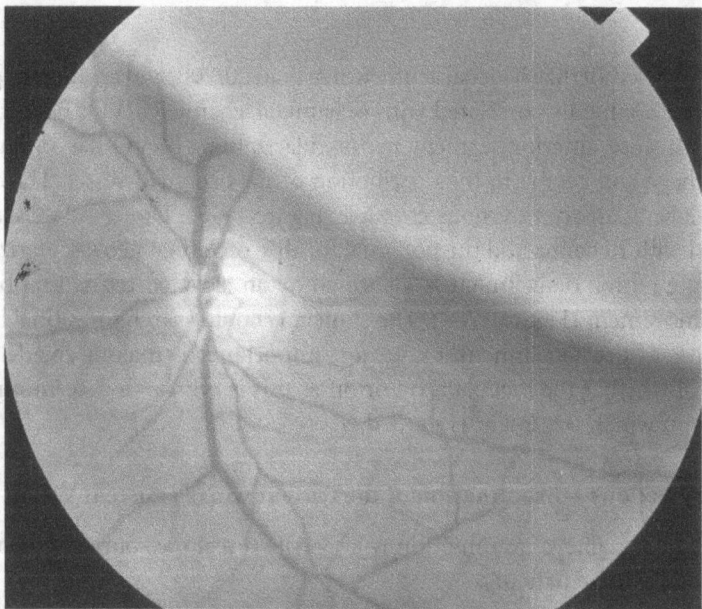

Figure 17–8. Macula-off retinal detachment that developed acutely in this 70-year-old male patient.

MANAGEMENT

The immediate treatment of patients with acute, persistent vision loss is dependent upon the results of the ophthalmic examination. Some causes may be amenable to treatment and the optometrist must first respond to the acute presentation in the hopes of restoring some or all of the lost vision. The patient may also require extensive medical evaluation to determine the underlying cause of the condition.

Vitreous

Patients with vitreous hemorrhage will often present with an accompanying medical diagnosis, usually diabetes. Patients with an unknown medical history need to be evaluated for the presence of conditions that may cause disc or retinal neovascularization: diabetes, central retinal vein occlusion, central retinal artery occlusion, ocular ischemic syndrome, sickle cell disease. The risk of vitreous hemorrhage in patients with CRVO, CRAO, or the ocular ischemic syndrome is not high because these conditions lead to anterior segment neovascularization more often than neovascularization of the disc or retina. Vitreous hemorrhage can also be associated with retinal tear/detachment so this must also be investigated. Usually, the extent of the hemorrhage will not be as extensive with a retinal break as it is with hemorrhage from neovascularization.

> *Search for a systemic illness or retinal tear in patients with vitreous hemorrhage.*

The management of the vitreous hemorrhage itself may depend upon the cause of the hemorrhage. For patients with diabetes, the Diabetic Retinopathy Vitrectomy Study (DRVS) tells us that prompt vitrectomy is indicated in patients with Type 1 diabetes or in those with poor vision in the opposite eye. A vitreoretinal specialist skilled in the management of diabetic retinopathy should determine the timing of vitrectomy in patients with diabetes. Vitrectomy in patients with vitreous hemorrhage from other causes is dependent on the nature of the condition and should be managed in consultation with the vitreoretinal surgeon.

> *Comanage patients with vitreous hemorrhage with a vitreoretinal specialist.*

Patients with vitritis need to be evaluated for conditions that cause posterior segment inflammation. Infectious conditions should be ruled out with VDRL and FTA-ABS for syphilis, toxoplasmosis titers, skin tests for tuberculosis, and titers for Lyme or toxoplasmosis infection. Inflammatory disease can be investigated by ordering nonspecific tests, such as ESR and C-reactive protein, or more specific ones, such as angiotensin converting enzyme (ACE) for sarcoidosis. Endophthalmitis must be excluded in patients who have had eye surgery or trauma.

Optic Nerve Disease

Optic Neuritis

The care of patients with acute optic neuritis is complicated by the relationship of the condition with multiple sclerosis (MS). The Optic Neuritis Treatment Trial (ONTT) tells us that patients with optic neuritis and two or more demyelinating plaques in the brain seen on MRI will benefit from steroid treatment as outlined in the ONTT (Table 17–3). (The ONTT steroid protocol is IV methylprednisolone 250 mg qid for three days followed by 11 days of oral prednisolone, 1 mg/kg of body weight. Oral prednisolone alone is expressly contraindicated.) The treatment benefit is prolongation of the time to development of clinically definite MS but this is lost by three years after the event. The interpretation of these data should be done with care and individualized for each patient and in consultation with a neurologist skilled in the care of the patient with multiple sclerosis.

> Use the results of the ONTT to guide management of the patient with optic neuritis.

Clinically, the utility of the ONTT results has been limited because of a lack of a treatment for MS. If the treatment benefit was lost by three years, was there any particular benefit in placing the patient on vigorous steroid treatment? Thankfully, in the last few years, three medications have become available that have shown promise in delaying the onset of MS or slowing its progression. These medications, Avonex (interferon B-1a), Betaseron (interferon B-1b), and Copaxone (glutarimer acetate), act as immune system modulators

Table 17–3 Management of Acute Optic Neuritis

- Promptly and accurately diagnose optic neuritis
- Order magnetic resonance imaging
- If 2 or more lesions consistent with demyelinating plaques, treat according to ONTT guidelines
  - ○ 3 days of IV methylprednisolone, 1 g/day
  - ○ 11 days of oral prednisone, 1 mg/kg of body weight
  - ○ NEVER TREAT WITH ORAL PREDNISONE ALONE!
- Consider treatment of those without MRI lesions if they require rapid visual recovery
- Refer to a neurologist for evaluation and treatment

in influencing the course of the disease. The CHAMPS (Controlled High-Risk Subjects Avonex Multiple Sclerosis) Study has shown that patients with a unifocal sign of demyelinating disease including optic neuritis will benefit from steroid treatment of the initial event as described by the ONTT followed by long-term use of Avonex.

In the past, practitioners have wrestled with whether they should share information about the relationship of optic neuritis and MS with their patients. However, with the advent of the Internet, patients can have information about this relationship in seconds. This, combined with the availability of treatment for MS, makes it essential that eye care practitioners discuss the relationship between the conditions and refer for MRI and treatment when appropriate (Table 17–3).

Patients with AION need to be evaluated for giant cell arteritis (Table 17–4). This evaluation may be nothing more than looking at the patient's birth date, as AAION is extremely rare in patients under age 60. Patients with giant cell arteritis may have constitutional symptoms such as headache, jaw claudication, neck pain, weight loss, fever of unknown origin, muscle and joint pain, and a general feeling of malaise.

> *Rule out giant cell arteritis in patients with AION.*

They may have a history of polymyalgia rheumatica. CRAO and extraocular muscle palsies may also be seen in GCA. A distinguishing characteristic between NAION and AAION may be the appearance of the noninvolved optic nerve. Patients with NAION have, on average, smaller cups and discs than patients with AAION.

The so-called "disc at risk" is a very small optic nerve with no cup, which increases the likelihood of developing NAION due to the crowding of nerve fibers and increase in ischemia seen in these nerves. The clinician should remember, however, that patients with "discs at risk" could develop AAION (just as patients without discs at risk can get NAION) so caution should be observed. Suspected giant cell arteritis needs to be evaluated promptly as the risk of de-

Table 17–4 Management of Ischemic Optic Neuropathy

- Promptly and accurately diagnose ION
- Rule out giant cell arteritis
  - Ask about constitutional signs of GCA
  - Order ESR, CRP, and other laboratory tests that might uncover GCA
  - Refer for temporal artery biopsy (referral can be made through the patient's internist, a rheumatologist, or a neuro-ophthalmologist)
- If GCA is not present or is not likely, rule out other causes of optic neuropathy by clinical impression, laboratory testing, or imaging
- If the diagnosis is NAION, there is no treatment

velopment of permanent vision loss in the opposite eye is significant. These patients require STAT measurement of Westergren erythrocyte sedimentation rate (ESR) and C-reactive protein (CRP). ESR greater than 47 mm/hour and CRP greater than 2.5 mg/dL have an almost 100% sensitivity for the diagnosis of giant cell arteritis. The clinician must keep in mind that approximately 20% of patients with giant cell arteritis will have normal ESR, so if the constitutional signs and clinical picture are such that giant cell arteritis is likely, then treatment for the condition should be begun to prevent catastrophic vision loss in the opposite eye. The gold-standard diagnostic test for GCA is temporal artery biopsy. Biopsy of the ipsilateral temporal artery with care to ensure that a diseased portion of the artery is biopsied is essential. The contralateral artery may need to be biopsied as well if the ipsilateral artery biopsy is normal but the level of suspicion for the disease is very high.

Treatment for AAION involves starting high-dose oral steroids to prevent vision loss in the opposite eye; 80–100 mg or more of methylprednisolone is typical. The steroid is slowly tapered as the ESR and CRP decrease. Some practitioners advocate starting treatment with IV steroid according to the protocols of the ONTT.

> *Treat AAION with high-dose oral steroids.*

The consultant neuro-ophthalmologist or rheumatologist should make this decision.

Management of patients with NAION is essentially ruling out other causes of optic neuropathy. No treatment has been shown to be beneficial for this condition. The Ischemic Optic Neuropathy Decompression Trial (IONDT) did show that a much higher percentage (42.7%) of these patients than previously thought improve on their own. There is some evidence that aspirin therapy may decrease the risk of development of NAION in the opposite eye.

Retina

Retinal vein occlusion is highly associated with a cardiovascular disease profile. Hypertension is most prominently related, particularly with BRVO, but a general assessment of cardiovascular health is warranted. The search for an underlying cause of CRVO is particularly important in younger patients, who may not have any predisposing cardiovascular conditions. These patients may have hypercoagulable conditions such as antiphospholipid antibody syndrome, hyperviscosity states such as multiple myeloma, macroglobulinemia, or increased numbers of blood elements as in leukemia (white blood cells), thrombocytopenia (platelets), or polycythemia (red blood

> *Search for underlying systemic conditions in patients with RVO.*

cells). The use of estrogens may be associated. Infectious and inflammatory conditions such as sarcoidosis or syphilis may also be related. Elevated IOP is a risk factor as it reduces perfusion pressure; lowering of IOP, if it is elevated, is indicated.

Both BRVO and CRVO can lead to macular edema. Macular edema from BRVO should be treated with grid laser treatment to the affected area provided the occlusion has been present for three months or longer, there is no hemorrhage overlying the fovea, visual acuity is 20/40 or worse and is stable or declining, and a good-quality fluorescein angiogram shows an intact capillary network around the fovea. Macular edema from CRVO, although reduced angiographically after grid laser treatment, is usually not treated due to the greater damage to the vasculature from this condition and poor prognosis for improved final visual acuity. Exceptions are made in some cases, particularly in patients younger than age 65.

> *Follow evidence-based NEI guidelines in the care of patients with vein occlusion.*

Neovascularization can occur from BRVO and CRVO as well. Ischemic BRVO, defined angiographically as an ischemic area of 5 disc diameters or greater, can lead to neovascularization of the disc or retina (NVD or NVE). Treatment involves scatter laser treatment to the involved sector at the first sign of new blood vessel growth. Prophylactic treatment is not indicated. Ischemic CRVO, angiographically defined by 10 disc diameters or more of ischemia, can lead to devastating neovascularization of the iris and angle and neovascular glaucoma. Visual acuity less than 20/200 with an afferent pupillary defect and large amounts of intraretinal hemorrhage at presentation can usually identify patients with ischemic CRVO without fluorescein angiography. Treatment is PRP (scatter) as it is with any proliferative retinopathy. Prophylactic treatment is not indicated. Patients with CRVO need to be followed closely following presentation for the development of anterior segment neovascularization, particularly if they have the afore-mentioned signs of ischemic CRVO. Monthly follow-up for at least six months with careful iris and angle examination is warranted (Table 17–5).

Urgent care of CRAO is the immediate attempt to re-establish circulation to the retina (Table 17–6). If embolism is suspected or there is a visible embolus, an attempt should be made to dislodge it. Digital pressure or pressure with a gonioscopic lens should be placed on the eye for 15 to 20 seconds and released. The sudden change in pressure gradient may release the embolus. This measure should be repeated until more definitive care can be provided. The use of oxygen, carbon dioxide, or a combination of the two may also be tried. One

> *Immediately attempt to re-establish circulation in patients with CRAO.*

Table 17–5   Management of Central Retinal Vein Occlusion

- Attempt to establish whether the occlusion is ischemic or nonischemic
  - ○ VA worse than 20/200, an afferent pupillary defect, and large amounts of intraretinal hemorrhage are associated with ischemia
  - ○ Fluorescein angiography can be performed to establish perfusion characteristics but is not totally necessary; hemorrhage may preclude it being performed
- Monitor monthly for 3–6 months for the development of iris or angle neovascularization
  - ○ Refer for PRP at the first sign of either of these
- Consider grid laser treatment for persistent macular edema, particularly in patients younger than age 65
- Refer to an internist for physical examination with particular attention to cardiovascular disease if the patient has not been receiving care
  - ○ In younger patients, consider other causes for the occlusion

---

hundred percent oxygen has been used to try to reduce or eliminate the profound retinal hypoxia. Carbon dioxide, because of its potent vasodilatory effects, may provide increased blood flow or help an embolus move downstream. The combination of the two, carbogen (95% oxygen, 5% carbon dioxide), may provide the best combination of hypoxia reduction and vasodilation. Carbogen is inhaled for 10 minutes every two hours for up to 48 hours. Anterior chamber paracentesis will rapidly decrease IOP, thereby improving retinal perfusion pressure. Lowering of the IOP by medical means will provide a similar but much slower effect. IV or oral acetazolamide in combination with topical antiglaucoma medications has been used. Although retinal tissue will survive without oxygen for only minutes, the practitioner should not give up in trying to re-establish circulation, as CRAO is often not complete. Circulatory improvements even hours after the event have been known to markedly improve final visual result.

Heroic measures are not indicated in the treatment of BRAO as these patients usually retain good visual acuity. In BRAO, embolism is far and away the most likely cause of the occlusion. Attempts to dislodge the embolus by pressure to the eye may be enough to dislodge the plaque.

The ultimate treatment of retinal artery occlusion is the determination of the cause of the problem. As BRAO is almost always embolic in nature, workup of the heart and carotid arteries is indicated. The heart is the most likely source of embolus that causes occlusion, so searches for conditions that cause cardiac thrombosis are indicated. These include atrial fibrillation, mitral or aortic valve disease, myocardial infarct, and car-

Search for the underlying cause of RAO.

Table 17–6 Management of Central Retinal Artery Occlusion

- Attempt to reestablish retinal circulation
  - ○ Digital pressure
  - ○ Oxygen, carbon dioxide, or carbogen
  - ○ Paracentesis
  - ○ Lowering of IOP by medical means
- Determine the cause of the occlusion
  - ○ Cardiovascular
    - ■ EKG
    - ■ Holter monitor
    - ■ Echocardiogram
    - ■ Carotid duplex scan
    - ■ MRA
    - ■ Angiography
  - ○ Other causes including infectious, inflammatory, etc.
    - ■ CBC
    - ■ ESR
    - ■ CRP
    - ■ Blood glucose
    - ■ VDRL
    - ■ FTA-ABS
    - ■ ANA
    - ■ ACE
    - ■ Antiphospholipid antibodies
    - ■ Clotting factors
    - ■ Chest X-ray

diomyopathy. EKG, 24-hour Holter monitor, and transthoracic or transesophageal echocardiography are indicated in the management of these patients in consultation with a cardiologist. Workup of the carotid arteries by noninvasive means with duplex scanning or magnetic resonance angiography (MRA) should also be performed to search for an embolic source and to uncover significant concurrent extracranial or intracranial carotid artery disease. As part of the general workup of these patients, or if other causes of occlusion are suspected, laboratory testing including CBC, ESR, CRP, blood glucose, VDRL, FTA-ABS, ANA, ACE, antiphospholipid antibodies, clotting factors, and chest X-ray might be included. In patients older than age 60, giant cell arteritis should be suspected, particularly if the patient has constitutional signs of the condition. Younger patients with retinal artery occlusion should be suspected of having a nonvascular cause of the condition and laboratory workup for another etiology should be intensified.

Patients with suspected choroidal neovascularization (CNV) require prompt fluorescein angiography to determine the presence, extent, and characteristics of the membrane. The angiogram should be acquired within 72 hours of presentation as choroidal neovascular membranes (CNVM) can extend very rapidly. Treatment of these membranes has been guided by the Macular Photocoagulation Study (MPS) for the last 20 years. The MPS is a National Eye Institute multi-center trial comparing laser treatment versus no treatment in patients with CNVM from AMD, POHS, or idiopathic causes. In the AMD arm of the study, membranes are considered extrafoveal (between 200 and 2500 microns from the center of the macula), juxtafoveal (between 1 and 199 microns from the center of the macula), and subfoveal. Membranes are classified as classic (well defined) or occult (ill defined) based on their fluorescein angiographic characteristics. Briefly, for AMD, laser treatment should be recommended for patients with classic extrafoveal and juxtafoveal membranes, and with caution in some patients with classic subfoveal membranes provided the patient is aware that he or she will lose vision immediately upon foveal laser treatment. Occult and partially occult membranes were not found to benefit from treatment. Treatment of CNVM from other causes was more amenable to laser treatment and provided a better visual result. Indocyanine green angiography and laser-guided treatment have been helpful in identifying occult forms of CNVM and have made laser treatment available to more patients with CNVM.

Fluorescein angiography should be performed within 72 hours in patients with suspected CNVM.

Unfortunately, laser treatment for CNVM in AMD still results in poor visual results or is not suitable for the majority of patients with this condition. Newer treatments, including photodynamic therapy, transpupillary thermotherapy, feeder vessel photocoagulation, submacular surgery, gas bubble tamponade, and medical therapy with antiangiogenic medications, have been or are being developed. Photodynamic therapy (PDT) has been approved for use in patients with subfoveal predominantly classic lesions. PDT works by laser-induced activation of an injected photosensitive dye. Verteporfin is the only such dye approved at this time. The activated dye, which has been taken up by the actively proliferating endothelial cells of the CNVM, leads to vascular thrombosis by free radical and singlet oxygen formation. Stabilization but not improvement of vision is the norm. The treatment is limited by the frequent need for multiple applications and by its cost. However, the advent of this treatment has given new hope to some patients with this disease. PDT is becoming the treatment of choice for subfoveal choroidal neovascularization.

Consider PDT for patients with subfoveal CNVM.

Transpupillary thermotherapy (TTT) has shown some promise in the treatment of subfoveal occult membranes. Submacular surgery aided by tissue plasminogen activator (TPA) might be useful for patients with macular hemorrhage if performed soon after the hemorrhage. Gas bubble tamponade with TPA may be as efficacious as surgery without the risk of going into the eye. Antiangiogenic medications may retard the growth of or prevent the occurrence of CNVM. A number of these medications are in development, including growth factor inhibitors, steroids, and nonsteroidal agents.

Ultimately, treatment of exudative AMD will lie with prevention that will include genetic manipulation and nutritional and life-style modification. A detailed discussion of the preventive treatment of AMD is beyond the scope of this book.

Macula-on retinal detachment requires immediate referral to a retinal specialist. If there is any question as to whether the macula is on or off, it should be considered on until proven otherwise. Before leaving the office, the patient should be told not to eat, as he or she will probably be under anesthesia the same day. The patient should be placed in the position that is most likely to prevent the macula from becoming detached (i.e., sitting up for an inferior detachment).

> *A vitreoretinal surgeon should see macula-on retinal detachment immediately.*

Macula-off retinal detachments do not have the same sense of urgency, but if they are fresh our recommendation is that immediate consultation still be made with a retinal specialist. Surgery may be delayed for a day or two, but the specialist should make this decision.

Surgery for long-standing detachments may be delayed for even longer periods or may be postponed indefinitely depending on the status of the opposite eye, patient health and wishes, and other factors that might affect the case.

Primary Actions—Management of the Patient with Persistent Vision Loss

- Patients with vitreous hemorrhage need to be evaluated for retinal detachment or tumor and for the underlying cause of the hemorrhage. Vitreoretinal consultation and management is indicated.
- Patients with optic neuritis should be managed according to the protocols established by the Optic Neuritis Treatment Trial and the CHAMPS study. A neurologist expert in the treatment of MS should be actively involved in the case.
- The management of ION first and foremost establishes whether or not the neuropathy is due to giant cell arteritis. Immediate ESR and CRP should be ordered with temporal artery biopsy when indicated. A

rheumatology consult should be sought. High-dose steroid treatment is essential to prevent the disease from occurring in the opposite eye. NAION requires no immediate treatment.

- The immediate management of retinal vein occlusion is the detection of the condition. The patient needs to be referred for cardiovascular workup and followed for the development of and potential treatment for macular edema or retinal or anterior segment neovascularization.
- Emergency management of retinal artery occlusion involves attempts to re-establish retinal circulation. Long-term management is the determination of the underlying condition.
- Discovery of choroidal neovascularization indicates referral for fluorescein angiography within 72 hours. Treatment will depend on the size, location, and angiographic characteristics of the membrane.
- Retinal detachment needs to be determined to be macula-on or -off. Macula-on detachment requires immediate referral for retinal detachment surgery to preserve central vision.

Flashes and Floaters

"Doctor, I've begun to notice flashes of light and many spots in front of my eyes."

SCOPE OF THE PROBLEM

One of the most common reasons patients present to the optometrist's office is because of flashing lights or floating objects in front of their eyes. Although isolated floaters are usually benign, these symptoms may indicate significant vitreoretinal pathology and should be taken seriously, particularly when a patient finds it necessary to present to or call the office on an emergent basis.

HISTORY

Although flashes and floaters often occur together, they can appear separately and we will first look at them this way.

Flashes (Photopsia)

The first determination to make is whether the patient has true flashes or pseudoflashes. True flashes are usually seen best in the dark, occur temporally, and are vertically oriented. True flashes indicate retinal stimulation, as the brain is only able to interpret retinal stimulation as light, even if the stimulus is not photic in nature.

Determine if the patient is seeing true flashes or pseudoflashes.

Pseudoflashes are perceptions of light that are really due to halos, glare, or photophobia. Halos may occur because of any ocular media change but are seen most commonly in association with corneal

Table 18–1 Flashes Not Attributable to
Vitreous Degeneration/Detachment

Pseudoflashes
   Haloes
      Ocular media change
      Corneal edema
   Glare
      Ocular media change
      Decentered IOLs
      Coated contact lenses
      Dirty or scratched spectacle lenses
   Photophobia
      Ocular inflammation
      Secondary to medication use
   Migraine
   Preretinal fibrosis (gliosis)
   Ocular inflammation
   Visual hallucinations

---

edema from elevated IOP. Glare is associated with lens opacities or any other media change, decentered IOLs, coated contact lenses, or dirty or scratched spectacle lenses. Photophobia can be due to ocular inflammation or be associated with glare. A number of drugs can cause photophobia as well (Table 18–1).

Scintillating scotomatous changes seen with migraine are also often reported as flashing lights. The differential is based upon the duration of the flashes: migrainous flashes usually last from 15 to 30 minutes whereas retinal flashes appear and disappear nearly instantaneously (Table 18–1).

An attempt to determine laterality should be made. Usually the patient is able to tell from which eye true flashes are emanating, as most true flashes are temporal and therefore on the same side as the eye that is having the problem. Migrainous flashes are usually hemianopic in nature and therefore are on one side of the body and not directly attributed to one eye. Of course, the patient may have difficulty making this distinction.

> *Ask patient which eye the flashes are coming from.*

If the patient is felt to have true flashes, the practitioner can assume that there is retinal stimulation. In most cases this is due to vitreous traction. The patient with acute-onset flashes consistent with retinal traction should be asked about the

> *Ask patients with acute-onset flashes about the presence of new floaters.*

presence and number of new-onset floaters (see below). Acute-onset floaters are usually due to vitreous degeneration.

The patient should be asked about whether the flashes are chronic, usually indicating an etiology different than vitreous traction. Preretinal fibrosis (gliosis), inflammatory disorders, and visual hallucinations can be associated with flashes (Table 18–1).

> Ask patient if the flashes are chronic.

Floaters

Although common, floaters can be indicative of significant vitreoretinal pathology if of sudden onset and increased number. The acute onset of floaters associated with flashes is indicative of vitreous detachment. If the floaters are few in number, the patient has probably had a benign posterior vitreous detachment. If the floaters are numerous and described as a curtain, cloud, or spider web of floaters, assume that a blood vessel has been torn and the likelihood of retinal tear has increased markedly.

> Ask patient if the floaters are few in number or numerous.

It may also be useful to ask the patient to describe the movement of the floaters. Floaters that follow eye movements precisely are usually due to opacities in the posterior vitreous near the retina; these are the common, benign floaters that practitioners hear about often. Floaters that overshoot the eye movements and rapidly return to the visual axis are vitreous opacities on the posterior surface of a detached vitreous. The patient can be assumed to have a posterior vitreous detachment (PVD).

> Ask patient about the movement of floaters.

Occasionally, a patient who has had chronic, benign floaters will be suddenly bothered by them and present acutely. For example, following cataract surgery some patients have a new appreciation of chronic floaters and present complaining about them. These patients deserve the same workup as any patient with new-onset floaters but the practitioner should be aware that the examination is likely to be negative.

Floaters that significantly worsen over time may be indicative of retinal bleeding, intermediate or posterior uveitis, or neoplasms such as reticulum cell sarcoma.

As the major determinant to be made in patients with acute-onset flashes and floaters is whether there is a retinal break, the history and record review should look for conditions that in-

> Identify risk factors for retinal breaks.

crease the likelihood for this to occur. These conditions include high myopia, lattice degeneration, and previous ocular (cataract) surgery.

Primary Actions—History of Flashes and Floaters

- Ask the patient to describe the flashes to determine if true flashes are present.
- Ask the patient if he or she has seen a sudden onset of floaters and, if so, to describe their number, appearance, and movement.
- Determine if the patient's history indicates that he or she is at high risk for retinal tear.

EXAMINATION

In almost all cases, the retinal examination will be able to determine the etiology and significance of flashes and floaters.

As always, visual acuity should be recorded. If visual acuity is reduced, retinal detachment or other active retinal or vitreal pathology should be suspected.

Pupillary reactions should be tested. If an afferent pupillary defect is present where none was seen previously, retinal detachment or other active retinal or vitreal pathology should be suspected.

Measure visual acuity, pupillary reactions, and IOP, and examine the anterior segment.

Slit lamp examination with attention to the anterior chamber should be performed. Inflammatory cells in the anterior chamber can indicate anterior segment inflammation or spillover of cells into the anterior chamber from retinal detachment, posterior segment inflammation, or neoplasm.

IOP should be measured. Reduced IOP in the setting of flashes and floaters may be due to acute retinal detachment or posterior inflammation.

Widely dilate the pupils and carefully examine the retinal and vitreous of both eyes.

Pupils should be widely dilated to allow careful examination of the vitreous and retina. It is essential that both eyes be examined to determine the status of the vitreous and retina in the noninvolved eye. The vitreous and retina should be examined at the slit lamp and with the binocular indirect ophthalmoscope.

The vitreous should be inspected for the presence of pigment (Schaefer's sign), blood, cells, and syneresis. The presence of a floating complete or incomplete glial ring of tissue (Weiss ring) near the disc is diagnostic for PVD. The vitreous detachment may be complete or incomplete. The relationship of the vitreous to the retina should be determined.

Look for signs of vitreous degeneration and detachment, and the presence of pigment, blood, or cells.

The retina should be examined carefully with the binocular indirect ophthalmoscope without and with scleral depression. The most important determination to be made is whether the retina has been torn or detached during the acute phase of retinal traction (Figures 18–1 and 18–2). In the case of retinal detachment, determine if the macula is attached or detached. Additionally, other causes of vitreoretinal traction, such as retinal tufts or meridional folds, should be sought out.

Carefully examine the retina without and with scleral depression.

If vitreoretinal pathology is not seen, other causes of flashes or floaters should be excluded (Table 18–2). Flashes may be seen in inflammatory chorioretinal disorders such as multiple evanescent white dot syndrome (MEWDS),

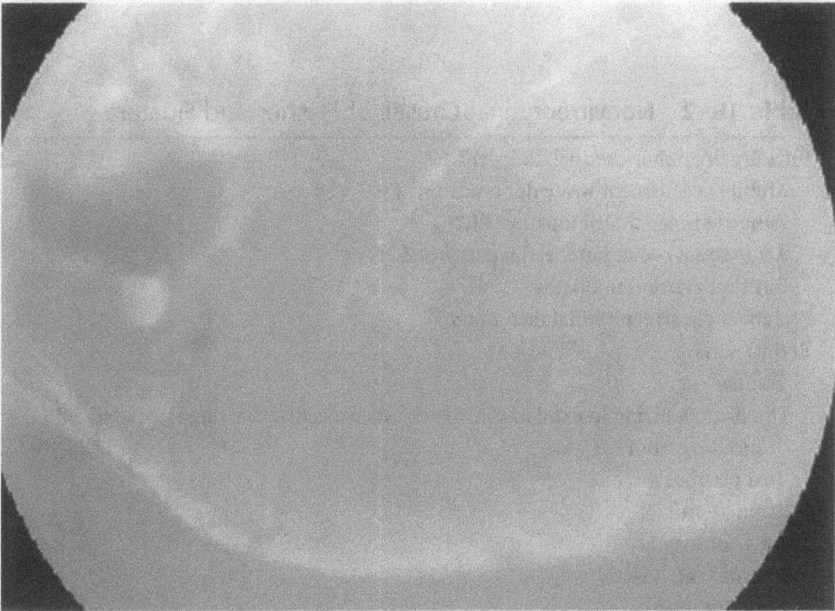

Figure 18–1. Peripheral rhegmatogenous retinal detachment following acute PVD.

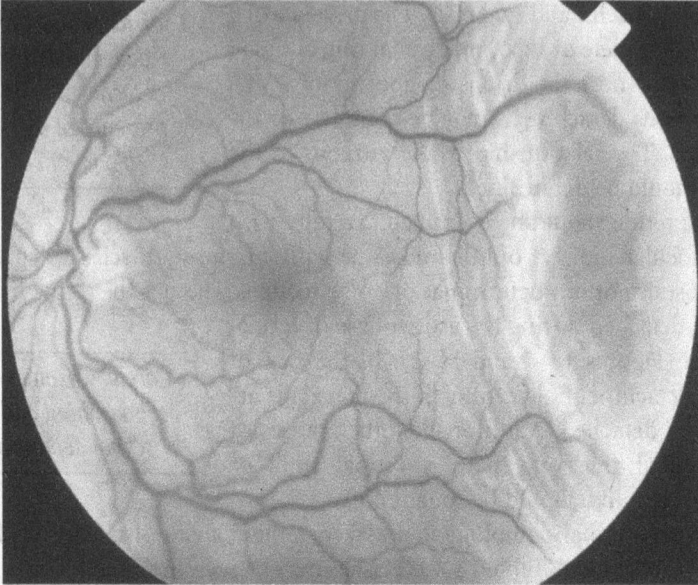

Figure 18–2. Macula on rhegmatogenous retinal detachment following acute PVD.

Table 18–2   Nonvitreoretinal Causes of Flashes and Floaters

Inflammatory chorioretinal disorders
   Multiple evanescent white dot syndrome (MEWDS)
   Punctate inner choroidopathy (PIC)
   Acute zonal occult outer retinopathy (AZOOR)
   Birdshot chorioretinopathy
Preretinal gliosis (epiretinal membrane)
Retinal scars
   Trauma
   Disciform scarring in exudative AMD or other macular scarring associated with
      bleeding from CNVM
   Toxoplasmosis
Inflammation
   Anterior uveitis
   Intermediate uveitis
   Posterior uveitis
Vitreal bleeding
   Vitreous hemorrhage from retinal neovascularization
   Breakthrough bleeding from choroidal neovascularization

punctate inner choroidopathy (PIC), acute zonal occult outer retinopathy (AZOOR), or birdshot chorioretinopathy. The prevalence of these conditions is low. Retinal scars from trauma or from exudative macular degeneration can contract and cause photopsia. Preretinal gliosis can also lead to

If vitreoretinal pathology is not found, look for other causes of flashes and floaters.

retinal traction and photopsia. Floaters can be seen in inflammatory conditions such as intermediate uveitis (pars planitis) in which vitreous cells accumulate near the ora serrata (snowbanking). Retinal neovascularization with bleeding into the vitreous can also lead to the acute onset of floaters.

Primary Actions—Examination of the Patient with Flashes and Floaters

- By far, the most important action taken is to determine whether a retinal tear or detachment is present.
- Careful examination of the relationship of the vitreous to the retina is needed to determine further actions.

MANAGEMENT

If the vitreoretinal examination does not show retinal tear or detachment, management will depend on the cause of retinal stimulation. By far the most common cause will be vitreous degeneration or detachment. Statistically, the prevalence of PVD is approximately equal to the patient's age over 50 years. That is, there is about a 60% prevalence of PVD in patients aged 60 years.

Acute, symptomatic PVD without retinal break requires careful follow-up. Approximately 25% of symptomatic PVDs are associated with retinal breaks. The risk increases to about 75% in those patients with associated pre-retinal or vitreal hemorrhage. Statistically, the patient is at greatest risk for the development of a subsequent break in the first month following the event. Therefore, the patient should be seen again

Follow acute, symptomatic PVD carefully until flashes stop. The risk of retinal break is greatest in the first month following onset.

in two to four weeks for dilated retinal examination. The patient is dismissed with instructions to return immediately if there is an increase in flashes or floaters or a decrease in vision. The follow-up examination will be the same as when the patient presented the first time. If the follow-up examination does not reveal retinal break, the patient can be seen again within the next six months provided the flashes have stopped (this indicates vitreous traction has stopped). Patients whose flashes are chronic but have normal retinal examinations need to be monitored for retinal break as long as the flashes continue. Monthly examinations should be performed until the flashes stop. The time between examinations may be lengthened if the frequency of the flashes decreases.

Educate patients about future risk of PVD in the opposite eye if it has not already had one.

Patients who have not had vitreous detachment in the other eye must be educated as to the likelihood of this occurring and the need for them to return for examination when it does occur. Patients who have had a PVD in the opposite eye are relatively free of risk and can be followed routinely.

Occasionally, the vitreoretinal examination will be normal yet the patient has symptoms of acute PVD. These patients probably have PVD in evolution and need to be followed the same way as patients with PVD.

Patients with retinal break following acute PVD usually need laser treatment to seal the break. These breaks have a high likelihood of proceeding to

Refer patients with retinal breaks following acute PVD to a retinal specialist.

retinal detachment because of retinal traction and the presence of liquefied vitreous at the site of the break. These patients should be sent to a retinal specialist for evaluation and treatment as soon as possible.

Immediate referral should be made for macula-on retinal detachments.

Patients with rhegmatogenous retinal detachment (Figure 18–1) may require urgent treatment. The status of the macula determines how quickly these patients need to be seen (Figure 18–2). Patients whose macula is still attached or in whom this is in question require urgent consultation with a retinal specialist. The hope is that reattaching the retina before the macula comes off can preserve central vision. If the macula is detached, surgery may be delayed for 24 to 48 hours.

If the cause of retinal traction is due to retinal tufts or meridional folds, the patient can be educated and followed. If the cause of flashes is an inflammatory disorder of the choroid and retina, the patient should be managed with a retinal specialist. Specific treatment of conditions such as MEWDS, AZOOR, PIC, or birdshot chorioretinopathy is outside the scope of this book.

The presence of retinal scars causing traction in one eye may guide the management of the other eye. A patient with a disciform macular scar from exudative macular degeneration in one eye, who has confluent drusen and RPE change in the contralateral eye, has about a 10% risk per year for developing choroidal neovascularization in the contralateral eye. These patients should be managed according to the guidelines outlined in Chapter 17. Scars from other causes, such as trauma, can typically be followed.

Primary Actions—Management of Flashes and Floaters

- If no retinal break is found, the patient should be examined again in two to four weeks to again rule out retinal break. If this examination is normal, the patient is educated as to the signs and symptoms of retinal break/detachment and seen again within six months. If this examination is normal and if the vitreous is detached in the fellow eye, the patient can be followed routinely. If the vitreous is attached in the fellow eye, the patient must be educated to return promptly with the advent of new flashes and floaters.
- If a retinal tear is found, the patient needs to be sent to a retinal specialist for laser treatment of the tear to prevent retinal detachment.
- If a retinal detachment is found and the macula is attached, the patient requires urgent treatment by a retinal specialist. If the macula is off, this treatment may be delayed for a short period.
- If other causes of retinal traction are discovered, they should be managed according to the protocols set for that particular condition.

Chapter 19

Postsurgical Care

In recent years, optometrists have taken on a greater role in the management of their surgical patients. In the majority of cases, this provides easier access and better continuity of care for these patients. Nonsurgical practitioners providing surgical comanagement must understand the normal postsurgical course and what constitutes a deviation from the norm. Especially important is the recognition of a postsurgical emergency and its appropriate treatment. Teamwork between the comanaging doctor and the ophthalmic surgeon are essential in ensuring that patients will receive the best care possible.

This chapter will look solely at postsurgical care and specifically at those conditions that require emergent care. Knowledge of preoperative management, surgical procedure, and normal postoperative appearance is important in the postoperative care of the patient but is outside the scope of this book.

GENERAL ANTERIOR SEGMENT SURGICAL CONSIDERATIONS

Similar postoperative complications are associated with cataract, cornea, and glaucoma surgery. Specific complications will be pointed out when appropriate.

Examination of the postoperative patient should be done systematically with emphasis on the recognition of high-risk problems such as endophthalmitis or wound leaks. The patient should be asked about changes in vision, increasing pain, uncharacteristic redness or discharge, and whether he or she is taking the medications appropriately. The clinical examination should focus on five "I's": infection, inflammation, incision, what is intrinsic

> *Systematically examine postop patients. Ask about changes in vision, increasing pain, uncharacteristic redness or discharge, and appropriate medication use.*

Table 19–1 Systematic Workup of Postsurgical Patients

History
- Change in vision
- Pain
- Discharge
- Redness
- Appropriate use of medications

Examination
- Visual acuity
- Pupils
  - ○ Reactivity
  - ○ Shape
- Incision
  - ○ Wound leak
  - ○ Sutures
- Infection
  - ○ Discharge
  - ○ Redness
- Inflammation
  - ○ Anterior chamber
  - ○ Corneal folds
- IOP
- Intrinsic to the case
  - ○ Particular characteristics of the surgery

In examining postop patients, think about five "I's" of follow-up.

to the case, and *IOP*.* Keeping this principle in mind should ensure that the practitioner would not overlook important aspects of the postoperative management (Table 19–1).

ENDOPHTHALMITIS

The most devastating complication associated with intraocular surgery is endophthalmitis. Endophthalmitis, usually caused by infection, is inflammation of all of the chambers within the eye. About two-thirds of all cases of endophthalmitis follow ocular surgery and the great majority of these are of bacterial origin.

---

*Per David M. Krumholz, OD.

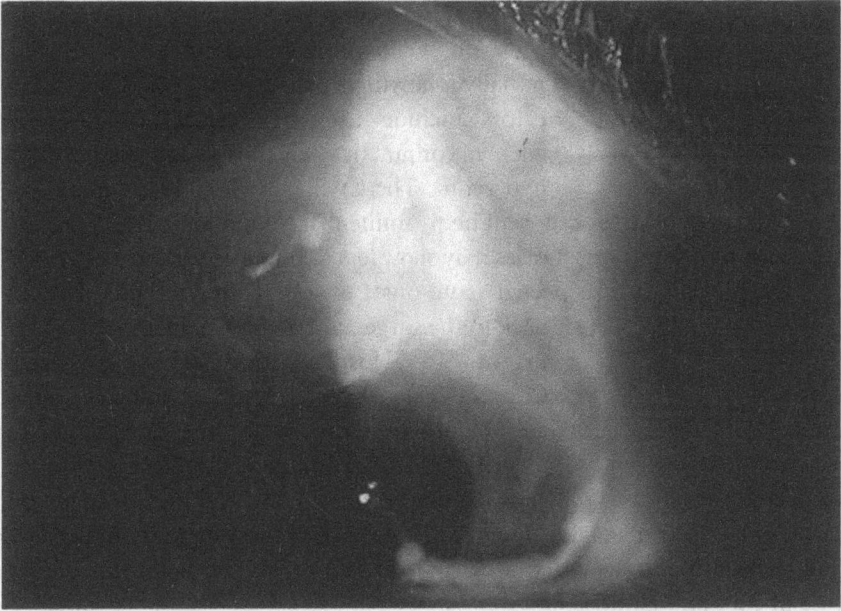

Figure 19–1.   Late-onset endophthalmitis (blebitis) in a patient who had glaucoma filtering surgery with adjunctive MMC two years earlier.

Most cases of infectious endophthalmitis are due to *Staphylococcus epidermidis* or *Staphylococcus aureus*. *Streptococcus sp.* and *Enterococcus sp.* are other common Gram-positive infectious agents. *Propionobacter acnes* is associated with late-onset endophthalmitis following cataract surgery. Gram-negative organisms include *Pseudomonas*, *Hemophilus*, *Klebsiella*, *Serratia*, and *Proteus sp.* Fungal infection can occur and is associated with later-onset disease.

Endophthalmitis can be acute, subacute, delayed, or chronic. Delayed or late-onset endophthalmitis is associated with glaucoma filtering surgery, particularly with procedures using adjunctive antifibrotic agents (Figure 19–1). Antifibrotic agents 5-fluorouracil (5-FU) and mitomycin C (MMC), while increasing bleb success by fibroblast inhibition and scar prevention, also cause the formation of thin-walled blebs. These blebs become thinner over time allowing for a portal for entry of infectious agents into the eye. As stated above, late-onset endophthalmitis after cataract surgery may also occur and is often associated with infection with *Propionobacter acnes* or fungal infection.

Late-onset endophthalmitis is associated with glaucoma surgery using antifibrotics and P. acnes or fungi following cataract surgery.

Increasing pain, especially after a pain-free interval, is an important characteristic of endophthalmitis.

The most important clinical indicator of acute-onset endophthalmitis is increasing pain, especially following a pain-free interval. Other indicators include decreased visual acuity, eyelid edema, conjunctival chemosis, and conjunctival hyperemia. There will be cells and flare in the anterior chamber. Vitreal cells will be prominent in fulminant cases. Chronic, subacute, or delayed-onset cases may show less dramatic signs and symptoms.

The patient with suspected acute-onset endophthalmitis should be sent back to the surgeon or a vitreoretinal specialist for urgent care. Hospitalization is often required. Conjunctival culture, anterior chamber tap and culture, or vitreous tap and culture are required to identify the causative organism. Subacute, chronic, or delayed-onset cases may not require hospitalization and may be managed in-office by the comanaging doctor or surgeon depending on the comfort level and relationship of the practitioners. Great caution should be taken with any case of endophthalmitis.

Refer patients with acute-onset endophthalmitis.

In all cases, treatment consists of the use of antibiotics that provide coverage against both Gram-positive and Gram-negative organisms. Injection into the vitreous cavity following immediate vitrectomy is the best course of action for acute, severe cases. Vitrectomy allows for easier culture and removes large numbers of the infectious agent from the eye. The Endophthalmitis Vitrectomy Study (EVS) studied patients with postoperative endophthalmitis. It showed that immediate vitrectomy provides a better final visual outcome in patients who present with LP vision or worse. There was no difference in outcome for those patients with better vision between vitrectomy and standard medical care. Overall, 50% of infected eyes had final vision better than 20/50. Intravitreal steroid injection may be added in addition to antibiotic to reduce the damaging effects of inflammation within the eye (Table 19–2). No long-term studies have been done showing the efficacy of this treatment.

INFLAMMATION

Postoperative inflammation is an expected finding in the perioperative period with its magnitude differing from patient to patient and dependent on the type of surgery. Inflammation disproportionate to the surgery with marked pain and IOP elevation needs to be treated aggressively and may be associated with endophthalmitis. As with inflammation from other causes, aggressive treatment with topical steroids followed by slow ta-

Treat postoperative inflammation aggressively.

Table 19–2 Management of Endophthalmitis

- Notify the surgeon and determine course of action depending on severity of case
- Acute, postoperative endophthalmitis
  - ○ Vision LP or worse
    - ■ Vitreoretinal consultation for diagnostic and therapeutic vitrectomy
    - ■ Broad-spectrum antibiotic coverage via intravitreal injection
      - □ Vancomycin, 1 mg/0.1 mL
      - □ Ceftazidime, 2.25 mg/0.1 mL, or Amikacin, 0.4 mg/0.1 mL
    - ■ Topical fortified broad-spectrum antibiotic
      - □ Vancomycin, 50 mg/mL q1h
      - □ Ceftazidime, 50 mg/mL q1h
    - ■ +/– Intravitreal steroid injection
      - □ Dexamethasone, 0.4 mg/0.1 mL
    - ■ Topical steroid, e.g., prednisolone acetate, 1% q1h
    - ■ Long-acting cycloplegic, e.g., atropine, 1%
  - ○ Vision better than LP
    - ■ Vitrectomy not indicated
    - ■ Anterior chamber tap and vitreous tap and culture
    - ■ Treatment—same as above
- Delayed, subacute, chronic endophthalmitis
  - ○ In some cases, can be managed without hospitalization
  - ○ Aggressiveness of treatment dependent on clinical picture
  - ○ Treatment may include:
    - ■ Topical, fortified, broad-spectrum antibiotics as above
    - ■ Broad-spectrum intravitreal antibiotics as above
    - ■ Topical steroids as above
    - ■ Add antifungal intravitreal or systemic if fungal infection suspected
    - ■ IOL exchange if this thought to be the cause

per is usually the best management. If infection is suspected, the appropriate anti-infective should be added to the treatment regimen.

HYPHEMA

Perioperative hyphema associated with surgical trauma is usually not problematic and blood typically resorbs rapidly. The hyphema may not clear as quickly in patients with cardiovascular or hematological disorders.

Late-onset hyphema occurs from tearing of blood vessels at the wound site or from erosion of blood vessels by an intraocular lens. Displaced or poorly positioned posterior chamber IOLs may damage ciliary body blood vessels causing bleeding, although inflammation without bleeding is more common. Anterior chamber IOLs have been associated with the UGH syndrome—

uveitis, glaucoma, hyphema. Management involves control of inflammation with steroid drops and cycloplegia and reduction of IOP with aqueous suppressants.

POSTOPERATIVE CORNEAL PROBLEMS

Treat postoperative corneal edema with anti-inflammatories, control of IOP, and hyperosmotics.

Corneal edema is common following anterior segment surgery. Damage to the corneal endothelium with concomitant inflammation is typical. Control of inflammation and intraocular pressure, with supplementation with topical hyperosmotic agents for superficial edema, is required.

Keratitis in the form of superficial punctate stain or frank erosion or ulceration can be seen. Causes include medication sensitivity, operative damage, or, in rare cases, infection. Treatment includes artificial tears and ointment, antibiotic drops, pressure patch, or bandage contact lenses, as with other types of keratitis.

Treat postoperative keratitis by the same means as you would treat nonsurgically related keratitis.

SHALLOW/FLAT CHAMBER

The depth of the anterior chamber should be evaluated in all patients following ocular surgery. Shallow chambers can be graded according to a simple grading system: Grade 1 when there is peripheral corneal-iris touch; Grade 2 when there is pericentral corneal-iris touch; and Grade 3 when there is complete iridocorneal touch (flat chamber). The etiology and subsequent management of the shallow/flat chamber is dependent on whether the IOP is depressed or elevated.

In cases of flat/shallow chamber, determine if the IOP is elevated or low.

Shallow/flat chamber with low IOP is due to wound leak, overfiltration, cyclodialysis cleft, or choroidal detachment, or is induced by IOP-lowering medications (Table 19–3).

Wound leak is suspected in all patients with low IOP and shallow chamber.

All patients with shallow/flat chamber and low IOP should be suspected of having a wound leak until proven otherwise. Seidel testing should be performed on all patients with shallow/flat chamber and low IOP (Figure 19–2). If a wound leak is

Table 19–3 Differential Diagnosis of Shallow/Flat Chamber

Low IOP
- Wound leak
- Overfiltration
- Cyclodialysis cleft
- Choroidal detachment
- IOP-lowering medications

High IOP
- Pupillary block
- Aqueous misdirection (ciliary block, malignant glaucoma)
- Suprachoroidal hemorrhage

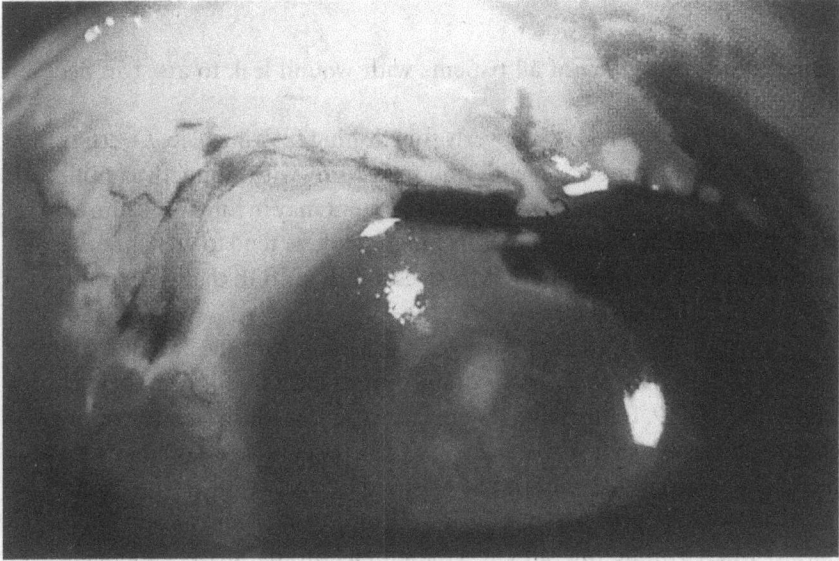

Figure 19–2. Appearance of a wound leak on Seidel testing.

discovered, management is usually conservative, as the majority of leaks will heal spontaneously. Treatment consists of pressure patching or bandage contact lens use, mydriasis, topical aqueous suppressants, and topical antibiotics (Table 19–4).

The majority of wound leaks can be treated conservatively.

Cyanoacrylate adhesive may be considered for large leaks. Larger leaks, nonhealing leaks, or those associated with dangerous sequelae (hypotony maculopathy, choroidal detachment) may require surgical intervention. The sur-

Table 19–4   Care of the Patient with Postoperative Wound Leak

- Identification
  - ○ Seidel Test
  - ○ IOP
  - ○ Status of the anterior chamber
- Notify surgeon
- Treatment
  - ○ Conservative—for majority of leaks
    - ■ Bandage contact lens or pressure patch
    - ■ Topical broad-spectrum antibiotic, e.g., fluoroquinolone
    - ■ Cycloplegia, e.g., 5% homatropine
    - ■ +/− aqueous suppressant
  - ○ Surgical intervention to repair leak

geon should be notified of all patients with wound leak to assist in decision making.

Overfiltration refers to an overly functioning filtering bleb. Overfiltration tends to occur in association with trabeculectomy with adjunctive antifibrotic agents and full-thickness procedures. Treatment may involve procedures to reduce the size of the bleb to reduce its function; these tend to yield poor results. Bleb revision is usually required to re-establish an IOP that does not have a detrimental effect on the eye.

A cyclodialysis cleft is an iatrogenic opening from the anterior chamber into the scleral space. Aqueous is drained from the anterior chamber, causing a lowering of IOP. If the cleft does not close spontaneously, treatment involves closure of a visible cleft with the argon or YAG laser or by cryotherapy through the sclera of a cleft that cannot be visualized.

Choroidal detachment or effusion (Figure 19–3) occurs as a result of hypotony whereby fluid migrates into the suprachoroidal space. Patients may be asymptomatic. Treatment includes topical cycloplegia and topical steroid drops (Table 19–5). Typical treatment would be atropine 1% bid and prednisolone acetate 1% qid. Usually the detachment will resolve without any other treatment over the course of a few weeks. Nonresolving detachments, those causing significant anterior segment shallowing, or large, abutting detachments ("kissing choroidals") may require surgical drainage.

> *Most choroidal detachments resolve with conservative treatment.*

Medication-induced hypotony most commonly occurs after glaucoma filtration surgery without discontinuance of IOP-lowering agents. It occurs much less commonly following cataract surgery. Treatment is as simple as dis-

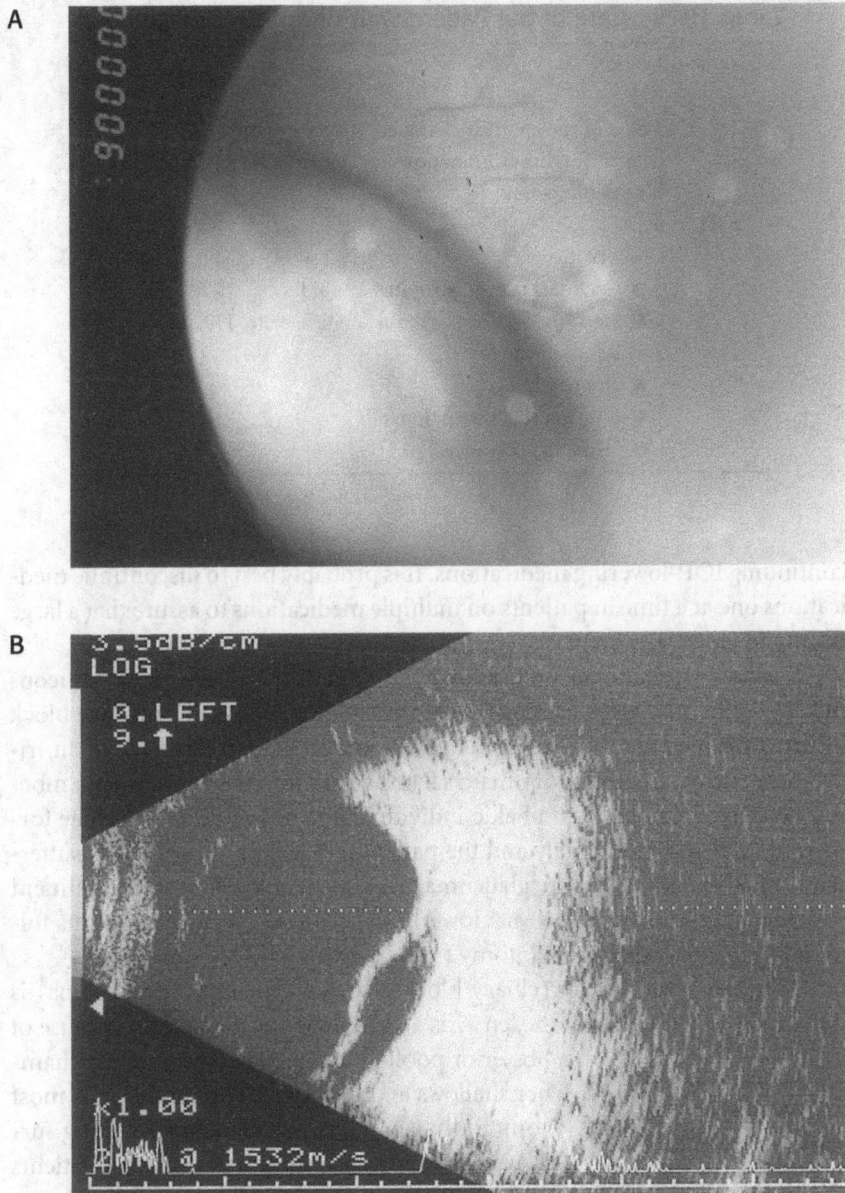

Figure 19–3. (A) Large choroidal detachments. (B) B-scan ultrasound showing choroidal detachment.

Table 19–5 Care of the Patient with Choroidal Detachment

- Identification
  - ○ IOP
  - ○ Status of the anterior chamber
  - ○ Dilated fundus examination
  - ○ B-scan ultrasound
- Treatment
  - ○ Conservative
    - ■ Cycloplegia, e.g., atropine, 1% bid
    - ■ Steroid drops, e.g., prednisolone acetate, 1% qid
  - ○ Surgical drainage for:
    - ■ Nonresolving
    - ■ Causing shallow chamber
    - ■ "Kissing choroidals"

continuing IOP-lowering medications. It is probably best to discontinue medications one at a time in patients on multiple medications to assure that a large IOP spike does not occur.

Shallow/flat chamber with high IOP is due to pupillary block, aqueous misdirection, and suprachoroidal hemorrhage (Table 19–3). Pupillary block in the context of anterior segment surgery occurs due to blockage of an iridectomy site by inflammatory material or by rotation of an anterior chamber IOL. It may also occur in a phakic individual due to posterior synechiae formation. IOP will rise acutely and the patient will feel as if he or she is suffering from acute angle-closure glaucoma. Treatment is similar to the treatment of acute angle-closure glaucoma: lowering of the IOP by medical means followed by peripheral laser iridotomy (see Chapter 15).

Aqueous misdirection (ciliary block glaucoma, malignant glaucoma) is due to anterior rotation of the lens-iris and hyaloid-iris diaphragm because of posterior pooling of aqueous. The anterior chamber shallows and IOP rises. The condition is most commonly seen following glaucoma filtering surgery in patients with short axial lengths. Patients with suspected aqueous misdirection should be returned to the glaucoma surgeon for care. Treatment consists of hyperosmotics, aqueous suppressants, laser treatment, or surgical intervention.

Patients with aqueous misdirection should be returned to the glaucoma surgeon for care.

Suprachoroidal hemorrhage is an operative complication in which hemorrhage occurs in the suprachoroidal space, shallowing the anterior chamber due to posterior pressure. As an intraoperative or perioperative complication, it is not usually a problem that the comanaging optometrist must deal with.

ELEVATED IOP

Postoperative elevated IOP (Table 19–6) can be assigned to early-onset (six weeks or sooner postoperatively) or late-onset causes.

Early-onset causes include:

- Retained viscoelastic material—Viscoelastic material not completely rinsed from the eye during surgery can cause a low-grade inflammatory reaction and concurrent IOP elevation. Appropriate management of inflammation will result in resolution. IOP-lowering agents should be used when the IOP is markedly elevated or in patients at risk for optic nerve damage due to elevated IOP. Occasionally, the inflammatory reaction and IOP elevation will be severe and needs to be managed aggressively with frequent use of topical steroids and aqueous suppressants.

Postoperative IOP elevation needs to be treated aggressively with anti-inflammatory and aqueous suppressive agents.

- Hyphema—Perioperative hyphema and elevated IOP usually resolve without treatment other than normal postoperative management of inflammation and IOP.
- Inflammation—Most postoperative patients will have some degree of inflammation. Occasionally, the inflammation will lead to elevated IOP. Unless the IOP is markedly elevated or the patient is at risk, control of the inflammation is usually sufficient to lower the IOP. Increasing the

Table 19–6 Postoperative Elevated IOP

Early-onset causes
- Retained viscoelastic
- Hyphema
- Inflammation
- Lens particles
- Vitreous loss

Late-onset causes
- IOL-related problems
- Inflammation
- Peripheral anterior synechiae
- Ghost cells
- Long-term steroid use
- Vitreous loss
- Epithelial ingrowth

frequency of usage of topical steroid drops is often adequate. Aqueous suppressants can be utilized when needed.

- Lens particles—Lens particles released after surgery or after YAG capsulotomy can set up an inflammatory reaction and lead to elevated IOP. Control of the inflammation is the appropriate treatment with adjunctive IOP-lowering medications as needed.
- Vitreous loss—The significance of vitreous loss will be discussed below.

Late-onset IOP elevation is due to:

- IOL-related problems—As stated previously, a malpositioned anterior chamber IOL can lead to damage to iris vessels with subsequent bleeding, IOP elevation, and inflammation—the UGH syndrome. Posterior chamber IOLs can damage ciliary body vessels leading to irritation, inflammation, and bleeding. In either case, inflammation needs to be managed with appropriate anti-inflammatory medications in combination with IOP-lowering agents when indicated.
- Inflammation—Chronic inflammation leads to IOP elevation due to deposition of inflammatory material in the anterior chamber or because of actual trabecular meshwork inflammation. Management is as previously described.
- Peripheral anterior synechiae—Peripheral anterior synechiae (PAS) can occur postoperatively due to chronic inflammation. Permanent damage to the angle may require filtration surgery to lower IOP if anti-inflammatory or antiglaucoma medications do not sufficiently lower IOP.
- Ghost cells—Ghost cells are red blood cell remnants that may remain in the eye after resolution of hyphema. Management of inflammation and IOP is necessary. Many patients require long-term topical steroid use to manage the chronic inflammation seen in these cases.
- Steroid use—A large number of patients will have IOP elevation in response to long-term steroid treatment. The elevation in pressure usually will not occur until at least two weeks after the start of steroid use although it may occur sooner in patients who have been treated with steroids previously. A change from a steroid more likely to raise IOP to one that is less likely to raise it is indicated. The typical clinical scenario is the change from prednisolone acetate or alcohol to fluorometholone, rimexolone, or loteprednol. Occasionally, topical nonsteroidal anti-inflammatory agents can be substituted for steroids with maintenance of good inflammatory control over long periods of time. In those patients whose IOP remains elevated, use of aqueous suppressants will be needed to control IOP. Discontinuation of anti-inflammatory agents is never

advised, as control of inflammation is mandatory in the postoperative patient. Adequate reduction of inflammation will eventually lead to IOP reduction in almost all cases.

- Vitreous loss will be described below.
- Epithelial ingrowth will be described below.

VITREOUS LOSS

Loss of vitreous is a relatively common but potentially problematic complication of anterior segment surgery. It occurs when the posterior capsule of the lens and anterior hyaloid face are damaged during surgery. Although it can occur in any patient, it occurs most often in patients who have had vitreous loss in the contralateral eye, those with weak zonules as seen in the exfoliative syndrome, in high myopes, or in restless patients who are unable to keep still during surgery. External pressures on the globe, as with suprachoroidal hemorrhages or with increased venous pressure, are also associated.

There are numerous complications associated with vitreous loss.

Postoperative complications due to or associated with vitreous loss are shown in Table 19–7.

- Bullous keratopathy—Vitreous release through the pupil and into the anterior segment can lead to endothelial touch and decompensation. Subsequent corneal edema can lead to stromal and epithelial edema with the formation of bullae. Treatment is via hyperosmotic agents, reduction of IOP, pain control, and anti-infectives and anti-inflammatories as needed. Irreversible bullous keratopathy requires surgical intervention via penetrating keratoplasty (Table 19–8).

Table 19–7 Complications Associated with Vitreous Loss

- Bullous keratopathy
- Epithelial ingrowth
- Inflammation
- Elevated IOP
- Retinal detachment
- Cystoid macular edema
- Endophthalmitis
- Vitreal bands and opacities
- Pupillary membranes
- Optic neuropathy

Table 19-8   Treatment of Bullous Keratopathy

- Hypertonic saline solution or ointment qid, e.g., Muro 128, 5%
- Mild topical steroid qid, e.g., fluoromethalone acetate
- Cycloplegia
- Broad-spectrum topical antibiotic qid
- Bandage contact lens or tarsorraphy
- Penetrating keratoplasty for irreversible cases

- Epithelial and fibrous ingrowth will be described below.
- Anterior chamber inflammation—Inflammatory reaction in the anterior segment occurs because of surgical trauma. Patients with vitreous loss typically have more complicated surgeries and therefore have greater amounts of inflammation.
- Elevated IOP—Eyes with greater amounts of inflammation are at greater risk for IOP spikes. As stated above, eyes with vitreous loss usually have more complicated surgeries and thus are at greater risk for postoperative IOP elevation.
- Retinal detachment—whenever the vitreous moves forward in the eye and therefore away from the retina, there is a greater risk of retinal traction and subsequent retinal tear and detachment. Eyes at greatest risk are those with the greatest amount of vitreoretinal traction, particularly high myopes, those with lattice degeneration, and those who have had a tractional tear or detachment in the opposite eye.
- Cystoid macular edema (CME)—see below.
- Endophthalmitis—Patients with complicated ocular surgery have a greater risk of endophthalmitis probably because of the greater amount of time the eye is open and exposed. Management of endophthalmitis was discussed earlier in the chapter.

EPITHELIAL INGROWTH

Poor wound apposition can lead to ingrowth of tissue through the wound site into the anterior chamber. As this tissue is in a place in which it does not belong, complications can occur.

Epithelial ingrowth should be managed in concert with the ophthalmic surgeon.

Epithelial ingrowth (downgrowth) is a rare but devastating complication associated with poor wound apposition and low IOP. An unhealthy endothelium that is unable to prevent the epithelium from encroaching is also related. A well-defined gray line is noted on the posterior cornea or on the surface of the iris. Progressive shallowing of the anterior chamber, inflammation, and elevated IOP are seen. Treatment is complicated and should be done in concert with the ophthalmic surgeon.

POSTERIOR SEGMENT COMPLICATIONS

- Cystoid macular edema (CME) can be seen following any anterior segment surgery, but is most commonly seen after complicated procedures with vitreous loss. It is seen less frequently since the advent of extracapsular cataract surgery and smaller wounds. CME was a common complication of intracapsular extraction; its presence following this procedure was termed the Irvine-Gass syndrome. CME should be suspected in any postsurgical patient with unexplained reduction of visual acuity. The forward movement of the vitreous leads to tractional forces on the macula and leakage of blood vessels. CME is a condition in which the perimacular capillaries leak fluid into the macular region, particularly Henle's layer. The anatomy of Henle's layer is such that the fluid accumulates in a cystoid pattern that is evident on fluorescein angiography. The macula and posterior pole may appear elevated or the condition may only be detected on fluorescein angiography. The majority of cases are self-limited but if vision is significantly decreased or not improving, treatment is indicated. Treatment consists of topical steroids, topical NSAIDs, or both. The trend today is toward the use of prednisolone acetate or alcohol qid and topical ketorolac qid. Nonclearing CME may require oral steroid (e.g., prednisone, 40 mg po qd for 2 weeks), oral NSAIDs (e.g., indomethacin, 25 mg po tid for 6 weeks), or sub-Tenon's steroid injection of triamcinolone acetonide.

> *Most cases of CME are self-limited. If treatment is needed, topical ketorolac qid and topical prednisolone qid are usually effective.*

- Hypotony maculopathy occurs in some individuals as a result of chronic or subacute hypotony. Very low IOP can lead to inward collapse of the scleral wall resulting in redundancy of the retina and choroid and chorioretinal wrinkling. These folds are the primary cause of reduced vision. Hypotony maculopathy, as well as progressive cataracts, inflammation, and choroidal detachment, is associated with IOPs lower than 4 mmHg. Treatment is aimed at the cause of the hypotony, for example, treating a wound leak. The best treatment is preventive: tight closure of sutures to prevent wound leaks and appropriate concentration of antimetabolites to prevent the formation of thin, leaking, or overfiltering blebs.

Patients with high myopia and lattice degeneration are at greatest risk for RD.

• Retinal detachment is a risk of any anterior segment surgery, particularly when there is vitreous loss. Patients with high myopia and lattice degeneration or other peripheral vitreoretinal abnormalities are at greatest risk. Treatment is as for any retinal detachment.

• Optic neuropathies, particularly nonarteritic anterior ischemic optic neuropathy (NAION), can follow anterior segment surgery. The probable cause is the elevation of IOP associated with surgery causing a change in perfusion to the optic nerve. There is a subset of individuals who are prone to developing this condition following cataract surgery. These patients are at risk for the same problem developing in the contralateral eye. There is no proven treatment for this condition.

COMPLICATIONS SPECIFIC TO TYPE OF SURGERY

Cataract Surgery

Postoperative complications following cataract surgery (Table 19–9) have diminished with the advent of smaller incisions and self-healing wounds. The major complications include infection (endophthalmitis), chronic inflammation with IOP elevation, and endothelial decompensation.

Patients should be examined the day following cataract extraction. It is expected that the patient will be relatively pain-free. There should be minimal mucopurulent discharge after patch removal. The examination should be concerned with visual acuity, the appearance of the eye and wound site, the amount of inflammation, the depth of the anterior chamber, the shape of the pupil, and the location and appearance of the IOL.

Qid topical steroid and qid topical antibiotic should be started on the first postop day following cataract surgery.

If all has gone well, patients usually use broad-spectrum antibiotic qid and topical steroid qid or antibiotic-steroid combination qid for one week. At the next follow-up, seven to 14 days post-surgery, the antibiotic can be discontinued if there is no sign of infection. The steroid is tapered by reducing frequency by one drop per week. Of course, this guideline is modified depending on the clinical appearance of the eye. Patients are usually next seen at four to six weeks postsurgery; spectacles can be prescribed at this time if the eye is not inflamed A dilated fundus examination should also be performed to ensure that the retina remains intact following surgery.

Table 19–9 Routine Postoperative Management of Uncomplicated
Cataract Surgery

Day 1
- Start postoperative medications
  - ○ Fluoroquinolone drops qid
  - ○ Steroid drops qid (or combination antibiotic-steroid)
- Instructions
  - ○ "Use the eye"
  - ○ Shield when outdoors or sleeping (extent based upon surgical trauma and presence or absence of sutures); minimal lifting
  - ○ Return if decrease in vision, pain, increase in redness, discharge

Day 7–14
- Medications
  - ○ Discontinue antibiotic
  - ○ Taper steroid by reducing frequency by one drop per week
- Instructions
  - ○ No specific restrictions
  - ○ Return if decrease in vision, pain, increase in redness, discharge

Day 28–42
- Medications
  - ○ Should be off medications
- Refraction
- Dilated fundus examination
- Plan for second eye

Anticipated findings in the immediate postoperative period include lid bruising and edema, ptosis, conjunctival injection and hemorrhage, corneal edema, anterior chamber cells and flare, and moderate elevation of IOP. Abnormal findings are deep pain, significant discharge, and abnormally high or low IOP. The practitioner must always be on the lookout for endophthalmitis in any postsurgical patient.

> *Deep pain, significant discharge, and abnormally high or low IOP are unexpected postop findings.*

Cataract surgery is the prototypical anterior segment surgery. The complications noted previously in this chapter as the common complications of anterior segment surgery are those seen most commonly in cataract surgery. Their identification and treatment have been discussed earlier.

A late complication of cataract surgery is capsular opacification. The posterior capsule clouds over due to the overgrowth of remaining lens epithelial cells that were not removed during surgery. This complication is now much less common as a consequence of improved surgical technique. Treatment is straightforward—clearing of the capsule using the YAG laser to perform a capsulotomy. Fortunately, complications of this procedure are rare and typically are limited to postlaser IOP spikes (see below).

Penetrating Keratoplasty

Corneal transplant, or penetrating keratoplasty (PK), is used most often to restore vision that has been reduced because of an opaque cornea, but may also be used for cosmetic purposes, to restore altered corneal structure, or to remove active corneal disease. The best prognosis for success is in conditions in which there is inactive disease with little vascularization, normal anterior segment structure, and normal IOP. As such, the best results are with keratoconus while the worst are with conditions marked by vascularization such as severe alkali burns or the Stevens-Johnson syndrome.

Day one evaluation of the post-PK patient should center on visual acuity, IOP, the presence or absence of pain, and the appearance of the graft. The prognosis is best if the IOP remains within normal levels. The patient should be on topical antibiotic and steroid; steroid taper is expected to take much longer than that seen in cataract surgery to control inflammation and reduce the risk of graft failure or rejection.

Steroid taper is slow following penetrating keratoplasty.

Primary graft failure occurs when the graft fails in the first 7 to 10 days following surgery. This is NOT an immune-mediated graft rejection; it occurs due to problems with the graft itself, such as poor handling or infection. Fortunately, this problem is rare today due to the sophistication of modern eye banks. Other early postoperative complications include wound dehiscence, high IOP, and epithelial defects. Wound dehiscence is treated as any wound leak. IOP must be controlled with aqueous suppressants to protect the corneal endothelium as well as the optic nerve. Epithelial defects are managed with artificial tears and ointments, topical antibiotic, and bandage contact lenses or patching depending on their severity. Postoperative endophthalmitis must always be considered as well.

Later postoperative complications are mostly concerned with graft rejection and the development of endophthalmitis. Graft rejection is marked by inflammation and corneal edema. Any post-PK patient presenting with new or increased inflammation and edema or pain should be treated as a graft rejection. The hallmark of graft rejection is the development of an endothelial rejection line (Khadadoust's line), a pigmented line composed of pigmented inflammatory cells. Patients with endothelial rejection have the most severe form of graft rejection and may present with pain, red eye, anterior chamber inflammation, keratic precipitates, and corneal edema. These patients should be treated with frequent (q1h) topical steroids and followed carefully for resolution. The corneal surgeon should be notified in all cases. Steroid taper must be extremely slow over the course of many months. Subepithelial infiltrates or epithelial rejection lines characterize less virulent forms of rejection. These are treated with less frequent applications of topical steroids.

Pain, red eye, anterior chamber inflammation, KPs, corneal edema, and an endothelial rejection line mark endothelial graft rejection.

Other postoperative complications include infection of the graft by the host, infection of the host by the graft, epithelial downgrowth, and retrocorneal membrane formation. Treatment of infection is with the appropriate anti-infective agent. Typically, infection is due to herpes simplex virus (HSV) infection that requires treatment with an appropriate topical or oral antiviral agent. Treatment of epithelial downgrowth has been described previously. Retrocorneal membranes are Descemet's membrane remnants inadvertently left in the eye at the time of surgery. This membrane may rest against the newly transplanted endothelium and cause focal edema, and potentially graft failure. If severe enough, this membrane may have to be removed surgically.

Postoperative astigmatism is a major determinant of visual success following PK. Many patients are left with significant amounts of regular or irregular astigmatism. Suture removal can begin at three to six weeks following surgery and can be performed so as to titrate correction of the astigmatism. If spectacles or contact lenses cannot adequately correct vision, then relaxing incisions, wedge resections, or refractive surgery is necessary.

Visual success of PK is often dependent on the degree of postoperative astigmatism and the success in treating it.

Glaucoma Surgery

Glaucoma surgery is associated with a higher rate of early and late-onset complications as compared with other anterior segment surgeries. The widespread use of antimetabolites, while increasing the success of trabeculectomy, also increases the prevalence of some of these complications.

As with other anterior segment surgeries, the visual acuity, wound site, presence of infection and level of inflammation, depth of anterior chamber, and IOP should be ascertained. Hypotony and shallow or flat anterior chamber are a particular problem and should be excluded in all patients.

Exclude hypotony and shallow/flat chamber in all patients following glaucoma surgery.

Suture management has allowed for the titration of the IOP in the immediate postoperative period. The surgeon can tighten the sutures at the time of surgery to reduce the risk of infection and prevent wound leak and hypotony. After about 7 days, the sutures can be lysed with the argon laser improving bleb function and lowering of IOP. Usually one or at most two sutures are done in any one session, with the impact on IOP and the wound evaluated before more sutures are lysed.

Late complications of glaucoma filtering surgery involve problems with the bleb itself. A "high-bleb" phase may occur approximately three to six weeks after surgery in which a diffuse, elevated bleb is found to have few surface microcysts and is limited by thickened subconjunctival scarring. Bleb massage, topical steroids, and topical aqueous suppressants can usually resolve the problem without further surgery.

Filtration failure can occur at any time following surgery. Scarring, an obstructed sclerostomy site, or an encapsulated bleb all can cause loss of bleb function and subsequent increase of IOP. Encapsulated blebs, or Tenon's cysts, are localized, dome-like, aqueous-filled elevations with overlying vascular engorgement and a thickened Tenon's capsule. These can be treated conservatively with massage, topical steroids, or antiglaucoma medications, but require needling of the bleb to rupture the capsule if elevated IOP persists.

Scarring is the major cause of filtration surgery failure.

Cataract is a significant postoperative complication of glaucoma filtering surgery. Cataract formation should be anticipated and must be considered in the overall management of patients undergoing trabeculectomy. Patients with significant cataract and glaucoma are candidates for a combined procedure.

Consider combined procedures in patients with significant cataract and glaucoma.

Chronic hypotony can occur after trabeculectomy. Hypotony is a more common occurrence since the advent of widespread use of antimetabolites. Chronic hypotony should be treated in cases of shallow/flat chamber, choroidal detachment, or hypotony maculopathy. Patients with low IOP without complications do not have to be treated but should be followed for the development of complications.

The increased use of antimetabolites in glaucoma surgery has led to the formation of thin-walled blebs with associated complications.

Thin-walled blebs are often seen after the use of antimetabolites. These blebs become thinner over time and may leak fluorescein. Blebs with significant leakage in association with low IOP should be considered for treatment as with any wound leak: pressure patch, bandage contact lens, antibiotic, or surgical intervention.

As with any other ocular surgery, endoph- | *Late-onset endophthalmitis*
thalmitis is a concern in patients with glaucoma fil- | *is associated with*
tering surgery. Bleb walls become thinner over | *glaucoma filtering surgery.*
time so later-onset endophthalmitis is more common following trabeculectomy than with other anterior segment surgeries. A more localized inflammation, blebitis, is also seen following trabeculectomy. A murky white bleb is seen surrounded by a very red eye (Figure 19–1). Blebitis may be a precursor of endophthalmitis. Treatment can be local but must be aggressive: frequent use of broad-spectrum antibiotics such as a fluoroquinolone q1h and cycloplegia. Worsening of the condition should lead to referral for treatment of full-blown endophthalmitis.

Anterior Segment Laser Procedures

The most common laser procedures used in the management of anterior segment conditions are laser peripheral iridotomy (LPI), laser trabeculoplasty (LTP, ALT), and YAG laser capsulotomy. Although technically dissimilar and indicated for different conditions, the postlaser treatment and complications are essentially the same.

All patients having anterior segment laser procedures will have some inflammation following the procedure. The amount of inflammation will depend on the amount of laser energy used and the individual response of the patient. Cells, flare, and pigment will be found. Treatment of the inflammation is topical steroid drops. Prednisolone acetate, 1%, qid for five days or higher doses tapered over one to two weeks is the typical postlaser management.

IOP spike following laser treatment was a major problem in the past. Since the advent of pretreatment with topical alpha-agonist drops (currently Iopidine, 0.5%, or Brimonidine, 0.2%), the frequency of posttreatment IOP spikes has fallen dramatically. Some patients will still have this complication, so all patients who have anterior segment laser procedures should have their IOP measured approximately one hour after the procedure. Patients with IOP spikes need to have their IOP reduced with aqueous suppressants before leaving the office and sent home with topical steroid and aqueous suppressant drops (Table 19–10). These patients should be seen the next day to ensure that the pressure is within a tolerable range.

Other complications of anterior segment laser procedures are uncommon. Laser peripheral iridotomy is occasionally associated with burns to the cornea, lens, or retina. Low-lying peripheral anterior synechiae may form in the angle following LTP but are usually not significant. Damage to the anterior nonpigmented TM can occur leading to poor IOP control and permanent damage to the TM.

Table 19–10 Postprocedure Care of the Anterior Segment Laser Patient

---

- Measure IOP one hour after treatment
- If IOP acceptable:
    - ○ Patient sent home
        - ■ Topical steroid drops q4h × 5 days or more frequent doses with slower taper
        - ■ Follow-up in 1 week
- If IOP unacceptable:
    - ○ Patient remains in office
        - ■ Topical aqueous suppressants and/or oral carbonic anhydrase inhibitors utilized until IOP at acceptable level
    - ○ Patient sent home
        - ■ Standard postlaser medications
        - ■ Follow-up in one day

SUMMARY

Optometric comanagement of laser and surgical procedures has allowed optometrists' patients the opportunity to receive postoperative care from their primary care doctor, improving access and continuity of care. Optometrists engaging in comanagement must remain well versed in all aspects of this care.

SUGGESTED READINGS

ADA Council on Scientific Affairs. Office emergencies and emergency kits. *The Journal of the American Dental Association* 133(3): 364–65, 2002.

Alexander LJ. *Primary care of the posterior segment*. 2nd ed. East Norwalk, CT: Appleton & Lange, 1994.

Alvey SD. Asthma emergency care: National guidelines summary. *Heart Lung* 30(6): 472–74, 2001.

American Optometric Association Clinical Practice Guideline. *Care of the patient with retinal detachment and related peripheral vitreoretinal pathology*. St. Louis: American Optometric Association, 1996.

Arffa RC. *Grayson's diseases of the cornea*. St. Louis: Mosby, 1997.

Augeri PA. Corneal foreign body removal and treatment. In *Optometry clinics*, Vol. 1, No. 4: *Anterior segment disease update*. Classé JG, ed. Norwalk, CT: Appleton & Lange, 1991.

Beck RW, Cleary PA, Anderson MM, et al. A randomized, controlled trial of corticosteroids in the treatment of acute optic neuritis. *New England Journal of Medicine* 326: 581–88, 1992.

BenEzra D, ed. *Ocular inflammation: Basic and clinical concepts*. London: Martin Dunitz Ltd., 1999.

Bennett J, Rosenberg MB. *Medical emergencies in dentistry*. Philadelphia: WB Saunders, 2002.

Burde, RM, Savino, PJ, Trobe JD. *Clinical decisions in neuro-ophthalmology*. 3rd ed. St. Louis: Mosby-Yearbook Medical Publishers, 2002.

Caffrey SL, Willoughby PJ, Pepe PE. Public use of automated defibrillators. *New England Journal of Medicine* 347(16): 1242–47, 2002.

Capucci A, Aschieri D, Piepoli MF, et al. Tripling survival from sudden cardiac arrest via early defibrillation without traditional education in cardiopulmonary resuscitation. *Circulation* 106(9): 1065–70, 2002.

Catalano RA. *Ocular emergencies*. Philadelphia: WB Saunders, 1992.

Catania L. *Primary care of the anterior segment*. 2nd ed. Norwalk, CT: McGraw-Hill/Appleton & Lange, 1996.

The Central Vein Occlusion Study Group. Natural history and clinical management of central retinal vein occlusion. *Archives of Ophthalmology* 115: 486–91, 1997.

Chern KC. *Emergency ophthalmology: A rapid treatment guide*. New York: McGraw-Hill, 2002.

Chernega JB. *Emergency guide for dental auxiliaries*. Albany, NY: Delmar/Thomson Learning, 2002.

Cummins RO, Hazinski MF. The most important changes in the International ECC and CPR Guidelines 2000. *Resuscitation* 46: 431–37, 2000.

Emergency Cardiac Care Committee, ECC and CPR Guidelines 2000. *Circulation* 102: I1–I85, 2000.

Emery RW, Guttenberg SA. Management priorities and treatment strategies for medical emergencies in the dental office. *Dental Clinics of North America* 43(3): 401–19, 1999.

Fraunfelder FT, Roy FH, eds. *Current ocular therapy*. Philadelphia: WB Saunders, 2000.

Friedman NJ, Pineda R, Kaiser PK. *The Massachusetts Eye and Ear Infirmary Illustrated Manual of Opthalmology*. Philadelphia: WB Saunders, 1998.

Fulcher TP, McNab AA, et al. Clinical features and management of intraorbital foreign bodies. *Ophthalmology* 109: 494–500, 2002.

Grambart S, Decker TL. Common office emergencies. *Clinics in Podiatric Medicine and Surgery* 19(1): 163–85, 2002.

Gresko SL. Medical emergencies in the dental office. *Dental Assistant* 69(5): 14–18, 2000.

Greven CM, Engelbrecht NE, et al. Intraocular foreign bodies—Management, prognostic factors, and visual outcomes. *Ophthalmology* 107: 608–12, 2000.

Handley AJ. Teaching hand placement for chest compression—A simpler technique. *Resuscitation* 53(1): 29–36, 2002.

Henderson, DP. Coping with asthma: The National Institutes of Health asthma guidelines. *Journal of Emergency Nursing* 26(1): 70–75, 2000.

Idris AH, Gabrielli A. Advances in airway management. *Emergency Medicine Clinics of North America* 20(4): 843–57, 2002.

Jones WJ. *Atlas of the peripheral ocular fundus*. Boston: Butterworth-Heinemann, 1998.

Kanski JJ. *Retinal detachment: A colour manual of diagnosis and treatment*. Boston: Butterworth-Heinemann, 1994.

Krupin T, Kolker AE, Rosenberg LF. *Complications in ophthalmic surgery*. St. Louis: Mosby-Yearbook Medical Publishers, 1999.

Laskowski-Jones L. Responding to an out-of-hospital emergency. *Nursing* 32(9): 36–42, 2002.

Limmer D, O'Keefe MF, Grant HD, et al. *Emergency care*. Upper Saddle River, NJ: Prentice-Hall, 2001.

MacCumber MW, ed. *Management of ocular injuries and emergencies*. Philadelphia: Lippincott-Raven, 1998.

Madonna RJ. Giant cell arteritis/polymyalgia rheumatica. In *Primary eyecare in systemic disease*. 2nd ed. Thomann KT, Marks ES, Adamczyk DT, eds. New York: McGraw-Hill, 2001.

Madonna RJ. Optometry and the carotid artery. *Journal of the American Optometric Association* 64: 390–402, 1993.

Malamed, SF, Robbins KS. *Medical emergencies in the dental office*. St. Louis: Mosby-Yearbook Medical Publishers, 2000.

Management of traumatic hyphema. *Survey of Ophthalmology* 47(4): 297–334, 2002.

Marenco JP, Wang PJ, Link MS, et al. Improving survival from sudden cardiac arrest:

The role of the automated external defibrillator. *Journal of the American Medical Association* 285(9): 1193–1200, 2001.

Mattei LC, McKay U, Lepper MW, et al. Do nurses and physiotherapists require training to use an automated external defibrillator? *Resuscitation* 53(3): 277–80, 2002.

Miller NR, Newman NJ. *Walsh and Hoyt's clinical neuro-ophthalmology.* 5th ed. Baltimore: Williams & Wilkins, 1999.

Modica, PA. *Neuro-ophthalmic system: Clinical procedures.* Boston: Butterworth-Heinemann, 1999.

Murrill CA, Stanfield DL, VanBrocklin MD, eds. *Primary care of the cataract patient.* Norwalk, CT: Appleton & Lange, 1994.

National Safety Council. *Pediatric first aid and CPR.* Boston: Jones & Bartlett, 2001.

Ophthalmology Clinics of North America—Mechanical Ophthalmic Injuries (Ferenc Kuhn, Guest Editor; Robert L. Stamper, Consulting Editor) 15(2), 2002.

Page RL, Juglar JA, Kowal RC, et al. Use of automated external defibrillators by a U.S. airline. *New England Journal of Medicine* 343(17): 1210–16, 2000.

Part 1: Introduction to the International Guidelines 2000 for CPR and ECC: A consensus on science. *Resuscitation* 46: 3–15, 2000.

Parver LM, et al. Characteristics and causes of penetrating eye injuries reported to the National Eye Trauma System registry 1985–91. *Public Health Reports* 108(5): 625–32, 1993.

Pieramici DJ, et al. Open-globe injury: Update on types of injuries and visual results. *Ophthalmology* 103: 1798–1803, 1996.

Ramaswamy K, Page RL. The automated external defibrillator: Critical link in the chain of survival. *Annual Review of Medicine* 54: 235–43, 2003.

Rhee DJ, Pyfer MF. *The Wills Eye Manual.* 3rd ed. Philadelphia: Lippincott Williams & Wilkins, 1999.

Rutledge D I. Cardiac emergencies in office practice. *Medical Clinics of North America* 53(2): 331–33, 1969.

Sapien R, Hodge D. Equipping and preparing the office for emergencies. *Pediatric Annals* 19: 659–67, 1990.

Tasman W, Jaeger EA. *Duane's ophthalmology,* Vol. 6. Philadelphia: Lippincott-Raven, 1998.

Thygerson AL. *First aid and CPR.* Boston: Jones & Bartlett, 2001.

Tuttle-Yoder J, Fraser-Nobbe SA. *Stat! Medical office emergency manual.* Albany, NY: Delmar/Thomson Learning, 1996.

U.S. Department of Health and Human Services. *Health, United States, 2000.* Hyattsville, MD: Author, 2000.

Vaughan CJ, Delanty N. Hypertensive emergencies. *Lancet* 356: 411–17, 2000.

Walsh TJ. *Neuro-ophthalmology: Clinical signs and symptoms.* 4th ed. Baltimore: Williams & Wilkins, 1997.

Weinreb RN, Mills RP, eds. *Glaucoma surgery: Principles and techniques.* San Francisco: American Academy of Ophthalmology, 1998.

Winbery S, Blaho K. How to prepare your office for medical emergencies. *Journal of Ophthalmic Nursing and Technology* 19: 164–65, 2000.

INDEX

Note: Page numbers followed by *t* indicate tables.

www.ingramcontent.com/pod-product-compliance
Lightning Source LLC
Chambersburg PA
CBHW011225210326
41598CB00039B/7313

* 9 7 8 0 0 7 1 3 7 5 5 3 5 *